European
School
of
Oncology

Monographs

Series Editor: U. Veronesi

D. Crowther (Ed.)

Interferons: Mechanisms of Action and Role in Cancer Therapy

With 8 Figures and 14 Tables

Springer-Verlag
Berlin Heidelberg New York
London Paris Tokyo
Hong Kong Barcelona
Budapest

Professor Derek Crowther

CRC Department of Medical Oncology
Christie Hospital NHS Trust
Wilmslow Road
Manchester M20 9BX, United Kingdom

ISBN-13: 978-3-642-76789-0 e-ISBN-13: 978-3-642-76787-6
DOI: 10.1007/978-3-642-76787-6

Library of Congress Cataloging-in-Publication Data
Interferons : mechanisms of action and role in cancer therapy / D. Crowther (ed.). p. cm. –
(Monographs / European School of Oncology)
ISBN-13: 978-3-642-76789-0
1. Interferon–Therapeutic use. 2. Cancer–Immunotherapy. I. Crowther, D. G. (Derek G.) II. Series: Monographs (European School of Oncology) [DNLM: 1. Interferons–metabolism. 2. Interferons–therapeutic use. 3. Neoplasms–therapy. QV 268.5 I61325] RC271.I461565 1991 616.99'406–dc20 DNLM/DLC

Softcover reprint of the hardcover 1st edition 1991

Typesetting: Camera ready by editor
Binding: J. Schäffer GmbH & Co. KG, Grünstadt
23/3145-543210 – Printed on acid-free paper

Foreword

The European School of Oncology came into existence to respond to a need for information, education and training in the field of the diagnosis and treatment of cancer. There are two main reasons why such an initiative was considered necessary. Firstly, the teaching of oncology requires a rigorously multidisciplinary approach which is difficult for the Universities to put into practice since their system is mainly disciplinary orientated. Secondly, the rate of technological development that impinges on the diagnosis and treatment of cancer has been so rapid that it is not an easy task for medical faculties to adapt their curricula flexibly.

With its residential courses for organ pathologies and the seminars on new techniques (laser, monoclonal antibodies, imaging techniques etc.) or on the principal therapeutic controversies (conservative or mutilating surgery, primary or adjuvant chemotherapy, radiotherapy alone or integrated), it is the ambition of the European School of Oncology to fill a cultural and scientific gap and, thereby, create a bridge between the University and Industry and between these two and daily medical practice.

One of the more recent initiatives of ESO has been the institution of permanent study groups, also called task forces, where a limited number of leading experts are invited to meet once a year with the aim of defining the state of the art and possibly reaching a consensus on future developments in specific fields of oncology.

The ESO Monograph series was designed with the specific purpose of disseminating the results of these study group meetings, and providing concise and updated reviews of the topic discussed.

It was decided to keep the layout relatively simple, in order to restrict the costs and make the monographs available in the shortest possible time, thus overcoming a common problem in medical literature: that of the material being outdated even before publication.

UMBERTO VERONESI
Chairman Scientific Committee
European School of Oncology

Contents

Introduction

Derek Crowther

CRC Department of Medical Oncology, Christie Hospital and Holt Radium Institute, Wilmslow Road, Manchester M20 9BX, United Kingdom

During the past 5 years, the European School of Oncology has introduced many new postgraduate educational initiatives. This series of monographs by experts in the field is based on a postgraduate teaching symposium on the interferons held in Venice, October 1991. These courses are designed to provide state-of-the-art information on important subjects in clinical oncology practice and research.

The interferons were the first human recombinant proteins to find a place in the management of human cancer and during the past 10 years the provision of genetically engineered material has allowed laboratory studies to determine many aspects of their biochemistry and mechanisms of action. Interferon alpha now has an established role in the management of patients with chronic granulocytic leukaemia, hairy cell leukaemia, myeloma, low-grade lymphoma, neuroendocrine tumours and some refractory solid tumours.

The chromosomal locations of the genes responsible for the production of the interferons and their receptors have been determined and many aspects of their physiological activity have been described including growth regulatory, immunomodulatory and antiviral effects. George Stark, an international authority on laboratory scientific aspects of interferon research working in the Imperial Cancer Research Fund Laboratories in London, has written the chapter describing the biochemistry of the interferons and their mechanisms of induction and response.

An international panel of expert clinical oncologists with pioneering experience in determining the clinical effects of the interferons has been formed to provide chapters on the mechanisms of action and clinical role in myeloma, lymphoid malignancy and neuroendocrine tumours. Dr. H. Mellstedt and Dr. A. Österborg describe advances in treating patients with myeloma including an update of their own trials in the Myeloma Group of Central Sweden. Dr. Ama Rohatiner provides an updated account of the role of interferon alpha in the management of low-grade lymphoma including the latest results of the UK study of chlorambucil and interferon alpha in follicular lymphoma. Kjell Öberg from the Ludwig Institute for Cancer Research in Uppsala, Sweden, is a pioneer in the management of neuroendocrine tumours using interferon alpha, and his chapter illustrates the advances made in treating these tumours using biological approaches. Dr. John Wagstaff from the University Hospital in Amsterdam has provided the final chapter summarising the latest advances in the use of interferons in combined therapy. It is clear that the use of recombinant interferon alpha has come of age and further applications using combinations of biological agents and cytotoxic agents in conjunction with interferon are only beginning. There is clearly considerable potential for improving our understanding of the ways the interferons produce their biological activity and enhancing their clinical effects.

The Interferons: Their Properties and Clinical Role - An Overview

Penella J. Woll and Derek Crowther

CRC Department of Medical Oncology, Christie Hospital and Holt Radium Institute, Wilmslow Road, Manchester M20 9BX, United Kingdom

In 1957, two scientists working at the National Institute of Medical Research in London discovered that virus-infected cells became resistant to secondary infection. Drs. Alick Isaacs and Jean Lindenmann found that influenza virus-infected chick embryo cells released a substance that conferred on cells of the same species resistance to a wide range of viruses. This substance was named interferon and is now known to be secreted in small amounts by most vertebrate cells when they are appropriately stimulated. Interferon was originally described as a glycoprotein containing about 150 amino acids. It is now known that several types of interferon exist with differing amino-acid composition and varying amounts of carbohydrate.

During the 1960s interferon was recognised to have antitumour effects in experimental systems but only in the 1970s were interferons derived from human leucocytes and lymphoblastoid cell lines made available for clinical trial. New molecular technology allowed the manufacture of recombinant human interferon alpha (rh interferon-alpha) in 1982 and subsequently rh interferon-beta and rh interferon-gamma became available. The introduction of these pure recombinant proteins permitted a more specific and quantitative approach to laboratory and human studies. A member of the interferon-alpha family was the first recombinant anti-cancer agent to be used in man. Despite this, as we enter the 1990s we remain unsure of the mechanisms regulating the most desirable attributes of the interferons and the best ways of exploiting them in the clinic [1].

Classification

Leucocyte, fibroblast and lymphoblastoid derived interferons have been classified as type I interferons. Leucocyte interferon obtained from the buffy coat was the first preparation to be used for its anticancer effects in man by Dr. Kari Cantell in Finland. Sendai virus was used to stimulate interferon production by the leucocytes. Lymphoblastoid

Table 1. Recommended nomenclature for the interferons

Nomenclature		Peptide sequences of recombinant interferons	
New	Old	Position 23	Position 24
IFN-N1	Lymphoblastoid IFN		
IFN-alpha 2a	Recombinant IFN-alpha A	Lys	His
IFN-alpha 2b	Recombinant IFN-alpha 2	Arg	His
IFN-alpha 2c	Recombinant IFN-alpha 2 arg	Arg	Arg
IFN-beta	Fibroblastoid IFN		
IFN-gamma	Immune IFN		

Table 2. Chromosomal location of interferons and their receptors

	IFN-α	IFN-ß	IFN-γ
Number of genes	24+	1	1
Chromosomal location	9	9	12
Receptor type	α/ß		γ
Chromosomal location of interferon receptors	21		6

interferon was obtained from lymphocytes transformed by the Epstein-Barr virus using Newcastle disease or Sendai virus stimulation. Immune or type II interferons are produced by T cells when they are stimulated by antigens or by mitogens. A subsequent classification has designated leucocyte interferon as interferon-alpha, fibroblast interferon as interferon-beta and immune interferon as interferon-gamma (Table 1). Lymphoblastoid interferon, a mixture of interferon-alpha and interferon-beta is predominantly interferon-alpha.

The chromosomal location for the genes encoding these interferons and their receptors is given in Table 2. At least 24 different interferon-alpha genes have been described clustered on chromosome 9 which encode 15 functional proteins. A high degree of homology exists between them (about 92%) and they are functionally indistinguishable. The interferon-alpha2 proteins differ from the interferon-alpha1 in having more amino acids and being glycosylated. Interferon-beta is encoded by a single gene on chromosome 9, close to the interferon alpha gene cluster. It is structurally related to interferon alpha (about 45% homology) and shares with it the property of acid stability. The 26kDa protein formerly known as interferon-beta2 is encoded by a gene on chromosome 7 and is now identified as interleukin-6. Interferon-gamma is a glycosylated protein of similar size to interferons alpha and beta but structurally unrelated, encoded by a single gene on chromosome 12. The alpha and beta interferons share a receptor of 110-130kDa but the interferon-gamma receptor is distinct. It has been cloned, and has a predicted molecular weight of 54kDa. The interferon gamma receptor appears to be G-protein linked and binding of its ligand activates a variety of intracellular signals including cAMP, inositol phosphates, Ca2+ fluxes and protein phosphorylation (see Stark, this volume). Some of the properties of interferon are summarised in Table 3.

Interferons alpha and beta are induced in leucocytes, fibroblasts and epithelial cells following viral infection and in response to double-stranded RNA, but interferon gamma is induced only by mitogenic stimulation of T cells and NK cells. Interferon beta is encoded by a single gene and its induction by viruses and double-stranded RNA has been the subject of detailed study. Positive and negative regulatory sites have been identified upstream of the interferon beta gene and transcription is enhanced by priming with interferon itself in some cell lines [2].

Table 3. Physical properties of the interferons

	Interferon-alpha 1	Interferon-alpha 2	Interferon-beta	Interferon-gamma
Number of amino acids	165-6	172	187	166
Glycosylation	No	Yes	Yes	Yes
Acid stable	Yes		Yes	No
Molecular weight	17-23kDa		~20kDa	~20kDa

Mechanisms of Action

After binding to specific cell-surface receptors, interferons induce and inhibit the expression of numerous genes. Some of the consequences are shown in Table 4. The interferons exhibit anti-viral, immunomodulatory and growth inhibitory properties. It is unclear which of these are responsible for the anticancer effects but it is likely that a combination of mechanisms is involved. Attempts to correlate clinical responses to the induction of 2', 5'-oligoadenylate synthetase, leucocyte guanylate binding proteins or NK cell activity have been unsuccessful. The antiviral and immunomodulatory effects of the interferons could stimulate host rejection of tumour cells and induction of MHC antigens. Stimulation of NK cell activity may be particularly important in this context, as may the enhanced expression of tumour-related antigens on the tumour cell surface. Other potentially important alterations in the host-tumour relationship could be mediated by the induction of a cascade of cytokines or growth factors, some of which may inhibit angiogenesis, haemopoiesis or epithelial proliferation, others may stimulate the immune system and induce inflammatory responses.

The interferons also have direct growth inhibitory effects, as demonstrated by the antitumour effects of human interferons on human tumour xenografts in nude mice. The human interferons do not bind to murine interferon receptors and the tumour regressions involved in this model system cannot be attributed to host interactions [3]. A majority of tumour cell lines are growth inhibited by interferons *in vitro*. The antiproliferative effects could be explained by inhibition of nuclear oncogenes, such as c-*myc* which has been reported to arrest progression through the cell cycle, although this does not appear to be an obligatory event [4]. Long-term treatment with interferons leads to differentiation and decreased expression of the transformed phenotype in some cell lines.

Table 4. Actions of the interferons

ANTIVIRAL	IMMUNOMODULATORY
Inhibition of viral attachment, uncoating, transcription, translocation + protein synthesis (α, β, γ)	Induction of - MHC class I antigns (α, β, γ)
Induction of - 2', 5'-oligoadenylate synthetase	- MHC class II antigens (γ)
- protein kinase	- β_2 microglobulins (α, β, γ)
- Mx protein (α, β) - resistance to influenza virus	- complement (α, β, γ)
- C56 protein - resistance to vesicular stomatitis virus	- IgG Fc receptors
- indolamine dioxygenase (γ) - resistance to toxoplasma	- tumour necrosis factor receptors
INDUCTION OF CYTOKINES	CELL REGULATION
Interferon-α (γ)	Macrophage activation (γ)
Tumour necrosis factor (γ)	Enhance NK cell activity (α, β, γ)
Interleukin-1 (γ)	Enhance B-cell proliferation + IgG synthesis (γ)
Interleukin-3 (γ)	Stimulate T-cell growth (γ)
GM-CSF (γ)	Inhibition of haemopoiesis (α)
Lymphotoxin, IP10 (γ)	Induction of thymosin B_4, leading to lymphocyte maturation (α, β, γ)
TRANSCRIPTIONAL INHIBITION	GROWTH INHIBITION
Oncogene expression, e.g., c-*myc*	Cytostatic (α, γ)
β-actin	Cytotoxic (α, β, γ)
Ornithine carboxylase	

Interferon Therapy

The demonstrated antiproliferative effects of the interferons on tumour cell lines *in vitro* and their anti-tumour properties in animal models led the way to clinical studies in man. In animal studies interferons used as single agents are capable of causing tumour regression and prolonged survival but they seldom achieve cure. The species specificity of the interferons was an added difficulty in preclinical evaluation and as is the case for other anti-cancer agents, animal model systems have not been good predictors of clinical outcome. Early studies were hampered by the use of impure preparations available only in small quantities. Despite this, anti-cancer effects were soon demonstrated in man.

Interferon preparations studied clincially include mixed interferon alpha subtypes purified from virus-stimulated lymphoblastoid cell lines (e.g., "Wellferon") and from virus-stimulated buffy coat cells, in addition to the single alpha subtypes produced by recombinant DNA technology (e.g., interferon-alpha2a "Roferon", interferon-alpha2b "Intron-A"). Natural human interferon-beta is unstable *in vitro* so the recombinant preparation in clinical use has serine substituted for cysteine at amino-acid position 17 (interferon-ßser). This compound is stable for prolonged storage periods.

A considerable amount of work is being carried out to identify structural determinants of biological activity of the interferons and new molecular species have been produced using insertional mutagenesis in an attempt to define a product with optimal anti-cancer effect. Clinical activity may vary with small stereospecific changes in molecular structure [5]. The glycosylation pattern of the different interferon products available in the clinic varies considerably and cannot be controlled by the manufacturing process. Its role in determining biological activity is unknown. Despite the large worldwide experience with interferons, their optimal dose and schedule of administration remain controversial (see Wagstaff, this volume).

Toxicity

The most commonly described side effect of interferon treatment is a 'flu-like syndrome of fever, headache, myalgia and fatigue. This begins within hours of interferon administration and typically resolves within 12 hours. For this reason many patients prefer to be treated in the evening. Nausea and vomiting occur occasionally but may lead to weight loss. These side effects frequently lessen in time in patients receiving continuous treatment. Transient elevation of serum transaminases occurs rarely. Hypotension has also been reported, particularly when high doses are used and may be related to vascular permeability problems with water retention. Bone marrow depression causing neutropenia and thrombocytopenia is more serious and can limit administration particularly when the interferons are used in association with cytotoxic chemotherapy.

Central nervous system toxicity including lassitude, depression and temporary memory loss are fairly common. Severe neurotoxicity may accompany high-dose therapy and may include encephalopathy, ataxia and cortical blindness [6,7]. Severe neurotoxicity is unusual at conventional doses but such changes can occasionally occur with interferon-alpha 3MU twice or 3 times weekly. As the interferons do not readily cross the blood-brain barrier, these effects are thought to be indirect and may well be related to the cascade of other cytokines released following interferon therapy. Cardiac changes have been reported in patients on interferon but it is not clear whether these are direct or indirect effects [8]. In view of the effects of the interferons on MHC antigen expression, patients have been closely monitored for the development of autoantibodies. A high incidence of thyroid autoantibodies have been reported with some patients developing overt hypothyroidism [9].

Clinical Applications

Hairy Cell Leukaemia

The first licensed application for interferon-alpha was for the therapy of hairy cell leukaemia. Since 1984, numerous clinical studies have confirmed its usefulness in this rare disease. Although highly active in hairy cell leukaemia, interferons do not cure the disease and prolonged therapy is necessary for the majority of patients. In a large multicentre study, 195 patients received interferon-alpha2b 2MU/m^2 three times weekly by subcutaneous injection for 12 or 18 months [10]. The overall response rate (complete responses + pathologic partial responses + haematologic partial responses) was 87% with significant improvement in anaemia, neutropenia and thrombocytopenia. Among 91 patients evaluable for the maintenance phase of treatment, relapse was more common in those assigned to observation only, but a further partial response to interferon was seen in about half of those retreated at relapse. Another study showed that after remission induction with interferon-alpha2a, approximately half the patients relapsed, at a median interval of 10 months and these relapses could be predicted by a persistently low platelet count on completing primary treatment [11]. Treatment is well tolerated if paracetamol is given prophylactically and the majority of patients with hairy cell leukaemia are symptomatically improved. Interferon-alpha therapy and splenectomy remain approaches of first choice in patients with this rare but potentially lethal form of lymphoid cell malignancy but combination with other forms of chemotherapy such as 2' deoxycoformycin are being evaluated.

Chronic Granulocytic Leukaemia

The clonal proliferation of Philadelphia chromosome (Ph') positive haemopoietic stem cells characterises chronic granulocytic leukaemia. The juxtaposition of the *bcr* and *abl* chromosome regions consequent upon the translocation t(9;22) (q34;q11) and the altered expression of a mutated tyrosine kinase appear to be key steps in the genesis of this malignancy. The indolent chronic phase of the disease persists for a median of 3-4 years before an accelerated phase and blast crisis supervene, the latter often being rapidly fatal. A variety of cytotoxic and biological therapies including interferon-alpha have been used to prolong and stabilise the chronic phase. Interferon-alpha is important in that it has the capacity to eliminate or significantly reduce the proportion of Ph'-positive cells in a substantial number of patients [12]. Ablative chemotherapy and bone marrow transplantation offer the best hope of cure but this high-risk strategy is impractical in many patients. Interferons may also prove useful as maintenance treatment following transplantation.

The first therapeutic studies were carried out using leucocyte interferon. In patients with chronic phase disease, leucocyte interferon-alpha 3-9 MU daily by intramuscular or subcutaneous injection induced haematologic remission in more than half the patients and cytogenetic remission in approximately one third. Similar results have been obtained with rh interferon-alpha. In a recent multi-centre trial of 107 newly diagnosed Ph'-positive chronic granulocytic leukaemia patients receiving rh interferon-alpha (5MU/m^2 s.c. daily), 55% achieved haematological remission (18% CR), median time to response was 6.7 months with 84% of responders, continuing in response beyond 1 year. Of 97 patients with cytogenetic follow-up, 19% sustained normal metaphases ≥50% and 13% achieved 100% normal metaphases (complete cytogenetic remission) [13].

Reports of cytogenetic remission in chronic granulocytic leukaemia must be interpreted with caution since many authors use only assessment of karyotype. Smaller quantities of abnormal DNA can be detected in these patients using more sensitive molecular techniques including Southern blotting and the polymerase chain reaction. Cytogenetic responses require more prolonged treatment than haematologic responses (median 9 months versus 3.4 months).

The patients most likely to benefit from rh interferon-alpha are those with early-stage, low-risk disease who have had no prior chemotherapy. A dose-response relationship has been described and the current recommendation is to start treatment with rh interferon-alpha at 5MU/m^2 daily and reduce only if side effects are unacceptable. The role of maintenance treatment continues to be the subject of clinical study. Although responding patients survive longer than non-responders, an overall survival benefit for interferon in chronic granulocytic leukaemia has not yet been demonstrated.

Interferons have also been used in the treatment of patients with chronic myelomonocytic leukaemia. The use of rh interferon-alpha2b (3-10 MU daily) reduced monocytosis in 8 of 10 patients but did not ameliorate ineffective haemopoiesis, hypergammaglobulinaemia or organomegaly [14].

Other Myeloproliferative Disorders

The success of interferon-alpha in controlling thrombocytopenia in chronic granulocytic leukaemia led to its use in other myeloproliferative disorders associated with thrombocytosis. Patients with polycythaemia vera, essential haemorrhagic thrombocythaemia, idiopathic myelofibrosis and other disorders have been treated with 5-25 MU interferon-alpha daily, with response rates of about 80% [15]. Long-term treatment is feasible and effective but it is not yet known whether therapy influences the risk of leukaemic transformation [16]. Although temporary responses have been observed in patients with acute myelogenous leukaemia, interferon-alpha has no defined clinical role in this condition.

Myeloma

Interferon-alpha has some activity when used as a single agent in patients with myelomatosis although the overall response rate of about 20% does not encourage its use for primary treatment. Interferon-alpha has activity in patients previously treated with cytotoxic chemotherapy and recent studies suggest that the combination of interferon-alpha and chemotherapy may be beneficial. A number of studies are showing benefits following the use of interferon-alpha in the maintenance of remission of patients with myeloma previously treated with chemotherapy (see Österberg and Mellstedt, this volume).

Non-Hodgkin's Lymphoma

Interferon-alpha has been found to have a useful role in the management of patients with low-grade B-cell non-Hodgkin's lymphoma. Up to one third of patients with previously treated follicular lymphoma will respond to interferon-alpha and a response rate of 40-50% in previously untreated patients was observed by Wagstaff and colleagues in Manchester using rh interferon-alpha2b [17]. The time taken to achieve a response is often longer than that seen following cytotoxic chemotherapy and no clear dose-response relationship has been established. Since alkylating agents are the most effective first-line chemotherapy for low-grade lymphoma, trials are in progress to evaluate whether interferon-alpha adds to their effects and several studies are being carried out to determine whether rh interferon-alpha is useful following remission induction (see Rohatiner, this volume). The interferons are less active in high-grade non-Hodgkin's lymphoma, although temporary responses have been seen.

The cutaneous T-cell non-Hodgkin's lymphomas, including mycosis fungoides and Sézary's syndrome, are indolent diseases which respond to ultraviolet, electron beam and X-ray therapy, in addition to cytotoxic chemotherapy and steroids. Trials of interferon-alpha (3-36 MU daily) have shown that this approach gives a response rate of about 65% [18,19]. Intermittent high-dose treatment (50 MU/m^2 daily) appears to confer no further advantage [20] but combinations with cytotoxic chemotherapy or retinoic acid derivatives may be of benefit [21]. Further study is required to determine the place of interferon in the overall management of T-cell neoplasia but rh interferon-alpha has been shown to be of benefit in some patients relapsing following primary therapy.

Hodgkin's Disease

Hodgkin's disease is frequently cured by modern radiotherapy and chemotherapy. New agents can therefore only be tested in relapsed patients who have been heavily pretreated. The finding that interferon can cause some disease reduction even in this setting suggests that it may be active against earlier stages of the disease [22]. It will be difficult to define a role for interferon in Hodgkin's disease because the success of conventional treatment demands that it be given in combination with existing regimens, so any benefits will be marginal and large collaborative studies would be required.

Neuroendocrine Tumours

Interferon-alpha has been successfully used to control symptoms of patients with a variety of neuroendocrine tumours and to induce regression of disease in some of these (see Öberg, this volume). Among 27 patients with carcinoid tumours treated with interferon-alpha 24 MU/m^2 thrice weekly, an objective response rate of 20% was seen, with reduction in 5-HIAA secretion in 39%, but at this dosage toxicity was troublesome [23]. In another study, patients treated with a lower interferon-alpha dose of 6MU daily fared better than those randomised to receive streptozotocin and 5-fluorouracil, with 72% improving subjectively and 50% objectively [24].

Other Solid Tumours

There is no evidence that any of the interferons used as single agents have a useful place in the management of patients with the more common epithelial cancers although some partial responses have been observed in a few patients. Renal cell carcinoma is poorly responsive to most forms of chemotherapy and radiotherapy. Phase I/II studies of interferon-alpha in advanced disease have yielded response rates of up to 27% but the overall response rate is only about 12% [25]. Others have reported useful responses in patients treated with interferon-gamma but the overall results are no better than those for interferon-alpha, and combinations of interferon-alpha with interferon-gamma have not been shown to be of any advantage. More encouraging results have been obtained with interferon in combination with interleukin-2 (see below).
A low but consistent response rate has been observed in patients with malignant melanoma treated with interferon-alpha. In 439 patients treated with interferon-alpha, an overall response rate of 15% was observed [26]. No clear dose-response relationship was seen in the range 5-50 MU/m^2 3 times weekly but the higher doses were barely tolerable and compromised patient compliance. Despite the low overall response rate, some durable remissions have been obtained particularly in patients with low-bulk and soft-tissue disease.
Early trials of interferon-alpha as first-line treatment in small cell lung cancer suggested a growth retarding effect [27]. In view of this, interferon-alpha is being studied as a maintenance treatment in patients responding to induction chemotherapy and radiotherapy in the setting of minimal residual disease. Although preliminary results have been encouraging, these studies have not yet matured [28].
There is evidence that interferon-alpha can have important effects on tumour vasculature because of its capacity to inhibit the proliferation of endothelial cells, smooth muscle cells and fibroblasts. Enhanced prostacyclin production by cultured endothelial cells has also been observed. Beneficial effects of treating patients with vascular tumours have been noted. Renal cell carcinomas are highly vascularised tumours associated with the production of tumour angiogenesis factors and in mice they are responsive to therapy inhibiting angiogenesis. Patients with metastatic renal carcinoma and haemangioendothelial sarcoma have responded to interferon-alpha. Useful responses have also been seen in patients with the benign but often fatal condition - pulmonary haemangiomatosis [29].

Regional Delivery

Although in most clinical studies interferon-alpha has been administered systemically, local and regional delivery have also been tested. The rationale was that high concentrations in the vicinity of the tumour would enhance the response rate while minimising the systemic side effects seen with intravenous, intramuscular and subcutaneous administration.

Intralesional injections of interferon-alpha in malignant melanoma and Kaposi's sarcoma have led to regression of disease in a high proportion of patients [30,31] but the significance of these responses in patients with disseminated disease is unclear. Topical interferon-alpha has also been used to treat carcinoma *in situ* of the vulva [32].

Intracavitary administration of interferon has been used in patients with malignant ascites and malignant pleural effusion and useful effects have been described [33]. The intraperitoneal administration of interferon-alpha in patients with ovarian carcinoma bearing small amounts of residual peritoneal tumour following chemotherapy has been associated with pathologically complete clearance of tumour [34,35]. The use of intraperitoneal rh interferon-gamma has also been attended by remissions in patients with minimal residual disease following chemotherapy [36]. The observation that there is a rise in antibody-dependent cytotoxicity associated with the use of intraperitoneal interferon suggests a potential benefit of combining intraperitoneal interferon with antibody therapy.

The instillation of intravesical interferon has been used in patients with carcinoma *in situ* or small amounts of transitional carcinoma of the bladder. A few partial and pathologically complete remissions have been described in this setting [37-39]. Recent attempts to deliver interferon-alpha topically to bronchio-alveolar cancers using aerosol inhalations have shown that this ingenious treatment is feasible but the response rates observed do not encourage further study [40,41].

Combination Therapy

Following the evaluation of interferons as single-agent therapy in a variety of tumours, several recent studies have investigated their place in combinations. The interferons alpha and beta have a common receptor which is distinct from that of interferon-gamma. In view of this, their combined use with interferon-gamma has been suggested in the hope that they might have additive (or even synergistic) effects. Although encouraging results have been obtained *in vitro* and in animal models, the results of clinical studies with combinations of interferon-gamma and either interferon-alpha or interferon-beta have been disappointing (see Wagstaff, this volume). The interferons are also being tested in combination with other biological response modifiers following optimistic laboratory reports. These include tumour necrosis factor and interleukin-2. Early studies with interleukin-2 alone were plagued by toxicity but lower doses and continuous administration have made combination therapy possible. Significant activity was seen in 95 patients treated by Rosenberg et al. [42] and 20-30% response rates in melanoma and renal cell carcinoma have been confirmed in studies from other centres. Improved tolerance to therapy has been obtained by giving both agents by subcutaneous injection on an outpatient basis [43].

Although interferon-alpha causes myelosupression, the agent can be successfully combined with cytotoxic chemotherapy. Animal models have predicted additive or synergistic effects in a variety of tumour types. Clinical studies have used combinations of interferon with chlorambucil, cyclophosphamide, cisplatinum, doxorubicin, vinblastine and 5-fluorouracil. In most of these studies the combination has added little to the effects of the chemotherapy alone, except toxicity [44]. A surprisingly high response rate has been reported by one group using a combination of rh interferon-alpha2 with 5-fluorouracil [45,46]. In this study, 32 patients with advanced colo-rectal cancer treated with 5-fluorouracil given by loading infusion and weekly bolus were treated using rh interferon-alpha2a 9MU 3 times weekly by subcutaneous injection. Partial responses were seen in 20 patients, some of which were prolonged. This interesting result requires confirmation in larger controlled studies. There is evidence that the administration of interferon-alpha alters the metabolism of 5-fluorouracil and the relationship between interferon and the metabolism of other anti-cancer chemotherapeutic agents is currently being studied (see Wagstaff, this volume).

Interferons and Infection

The interferons were first characterised as

antiviral agents, but they have not proved effective in the treatment of acute viral infections, although some studies have shown that they may inhibit their development if given before experimental infection. In contrast, they have proved useful in some chronic viral diseases including condylomata acuminata, laryngeal papillomatosis and hepatitis B [47]. Interferon-alpha has been shown to reduce viral carriage rates in chronic hepatitis-B but whether this will reduce the risk of hepatocellular cancer in these patients remains to be seen.

Preliminary studies in HIV-positive patients have suggested a possible role for interferon in suppressing the progression to AIDS. Larger studies are now being undertaken using interferon alone and in combination with zidovudine. Interferon also has a role in established AIDS, for the treatment of Kaposi's sarcoma. Response rates of 30% are seen, using interferon-alpha 20-50 MU/m^2 by subcutaneous or intramuscular injection. Interferon-alpha not only has an antitumour effect but also appears to suppress HIV replication. It is not yet known whether response predicts a better overall prognosis. The use of interferon-gamma in this condition has been disappointing.

Conclusion

The interferons are a group of natural proteins with defined activitites in a number of biological systems. The initial euphoria generated by testing these compounds as anticancer agents *in vitro* and *in vivo* has given way to cautious optimism born of mature reflection. The increasing knowledge of their mechanisms of action has led to innovative approaches in combination cancer therapy. Although the interferons already have a clearly established role in the treatment of hairy cell leukaemia and can be helpful in the management of patients with chronic granulocytic leukaemia, myeloma, low-grade lymphoma and neuroendocrine tumours, further study is required to define their place in the overall management of these conditions. The imaginative application of novel strategies promises further success in the difficult area of common solid tumours, including colorectal, lung and ovarian cancers.

REFERENCES

1 Balkwill FR: Interferons. In: Cytokines in cancer therapy. Oxford University Press, Oxford 1989 pp8-53

2 Goodbourn S: The regulation of ß-interferon gene expression. Sem Cancer Biol 1990 (1): 89-95

3 Balkwill FR, Mowshowtitz S, Seilman SS, Moodie EM, Griffin, DB, Fantes KH and Wolf CR: Positive interactions between interferon and chemotherapy due to direct tumour action rather than effects on host drug-metabolising enzymes. Cancer Res 1984 (44): 5249-5255

4 Mehmet H, Taylor-Papadimitriou J and Rozengurt E: Interferon inhibition of bombesin-stimulated mitogenesis in Swiss 3T3 cells occurs without blocking c-*fos* and c-*myc* expression. J Interferon Res 1989 (9): 205-213

5 Perez R, Lipton A, Harvey HA, Simmonds MA, Romano PJ, Imboden SL, Giudice G, Downing MR and Alton NK: A phase I trial of recombinant human gamma interferon (IFN-gamma 4A) in patients with advanced malignancy. J Biol Resp Mod 1988 (7): 309-317

6 Adams F, Quesada JR and Gutterman JU: Neuropsychiatric manifestations of human leukocyte interferon therapy in patients with cancer. J Am Med Ass 1984 (252): 938-941

7 Merimsky O, Reider-Groswasser I, Inbar M and Chaichik S: Interferon-related mental deterioration and behavioural changes in patients with renal cell carcinoma. Eur J Cancer 1990 (26): 596-6007

8 Cohen MC, Huberman MS and Nesto RW: Recombinant $alpha_2$ interferon-related cardiomyopathy. Am J Med 1988 (85): 549-551

9 Fentiman IS, Balkwill FR, Thomas BS, Russell MJ, Todd I and Bottazzo GF: An autoimmune aetiology for hypothyroidism following interferon therapy for breast cancer. Eur J Cancer Clin Oncol 1988 (24): 1299-1303

10 Golomb H, Fefer A, Golde D, Ozer H, Portlock C, Silber R, Rappeport J, Ratain MJ, Thompson J, Bonnem E, Spiegel R, Tensen L, Burke J and Vardiman JW: Update of a multi-institutional study of 195 patients (pts) with hairy cell leukaemia (HCL) treated with interferon-alfa2b (IFN). Proc Am Soc Clin Oncol 1990 (9): 215

11 Berman E, Heller G, Kempin S, Gee T, Tran LL and Clarkson B: Incidence of response and long term follow up in patients with hairy cell leukaemia treated with recombinant interferon alfa-2a. Blood 1990 (75): 839-845

12 Talpaz M, Kantarjian HM, Kurzrock R and Gutterman J: Therapy of chronic myelogenous leukaemia: chemotherapy and interferons. Sem Oncol 1988 (25): 62-73

13 Ozer H, Dear K, Testa J, Arthur D, Cooper R, Pettenati M, Ras K, Peterson BA, Schiffer C and Bloomfield CD: Prolonged administration of subcutaneous α interferon induces major clinical and complete cytogenetic remissions in untreated Philadelphia chromosome positive (Ph+) chronic myelogenous leukaemia (CML). Proc Am Soc Clin Oncol 1990 (9): 203

14 Catalano L, Majolino I, Musto P, Fragrasso A, Molica S, Cirincione S, Selleri C, Lucino L, DeRenzo A, Vecchione R and Rotoli B: Alpha interferon in the treatment of chronic myelomonocytic leukaemia. Haematologica 1989 (74): 577-581

15 Talpaz M, Kurzrock R, Kantarjian H, O'Brien S and Gutterman JU: Recombinant interferon-alpha therapy of Philadelphia chromosome-negative myeloproliferative disorders with thrombocytosis. Am J Med 1989 (86): 554-558

16 Gisslinger H, Ludwig H, Linkesch W, Chott A, Fritz E and Radaszkiewicz T: Long term interferon therapy for thormbocytosis in myeloproliferative disease. Lancet 1989 (1): 634-637

17 Wagstaff J, Loynds P and Crowther D: A phase II study of human rDNA alpha-2 interferon in patients with low grade non Hodgkin's lymphoma. Cancer Chemother Pharmacol 1985 (18): 54-58

18 Tura S, Mazza P, Zinzani PL, Ghetti PL, Poletti G, Gherlionzoni F, Motgagnani A and Criscuolo D: Alpha recombinant interferon in the treatment of mycosis fungoides (MF). Haematologica 1987 (72): 337-340

19 Olsen EA, Rosen ST, Vollmer RT, Variakojis D, Roenigk HH, Diab N and Zeffren J: Interferon alfa-2a in the treatment of cutaneous T cell lymphoma. J Am Acad Dermatol 1989 (20): 395-407

20 Kohn EC, Steis RG, Sausville EA, Veach SR, Stocker JL, Phelps R, Franco S, Longo DL, Bunn PA and Ihde DC: Phase II trial of intermittent high dose recombinant interferon alfa-2a in mycosis fungoides and the Sézary syndrome. J Clin Oncol 1990 (8): 155-160

21 Braathen LR and McFadden N: Successful treatment of mycosis fungoides with the combination of etretinate and human recombinant interferon alfa-2a. J Dermatol. Treat 1989 (1): 29-32

22 Rybak ME, McCarroll K, Bernard S, Lester E, Barcos M, Ozer H, Bloomfield CD and Gottleib AJ: Interferon therapy of relapsed and refractory Hodgkin's disease: Cancer and Leukaemia Group B Study 8652. J Biol Resp Mod 1990 (9): 1-4.

23 Moertel CG, Rubib J and Kvols KL: Therapy of metastatic carcinoid syndrome with recombinant leucocyte A interferon. J Clin Oncol 1989 (7): 865-868

24 Öberg K, Norheim I and Alm G: Treatment of malignant carcinoid tumours: a randomised controlled study of streptozotocin plus 5-FU and human leucocyte interferon. Eur J Cancer Clin Oncol 1989 (25): 1475-1479

25 Buzaid AC and Todd MB: Therapeutic options in renal cell carcinoma. Sem Oncol 1989 (16 suppl 1): 12-19

26 Legha SL: Current therapy for malignant melanoma. Sem Oncol 1989 (16 suppl 1): 34-44

27 Mattson K: Natural alpha interferon as part of a combined treatment for small cell lung cancer. In: Smyth JF (ed) Interferons in Oncology. European School of Oncology Monographs. Springer-Verlag, Berlin 1987 pp 25-32

28 Jett JR: Is there a role for interferon in the treatment of small cell lung cancer? Lung Cancer 1989 (5): 281-286

29 White CW, Sondeheim HM, Crouch EC, Wilson H and Fan LL: Treatment of pulmonary haemangiomatosis with recombinant interferon alpha-2a. N Engl J Med 1989 (320): 1197-1200

30 von Wussow P, Block B, Hartmann F and Deicher H: Intralesional interferon-alpha therapy in advanced malignant melanoma. Cancer 1988 (61): 1071-1074

31 Sulis E, Floris C, Sulis ML, Zurrida S, Piro S, Pintus A and Contu L: Interferon administered intralesionally in skin and oral cavity lesions in heterosexual drug addicted patients with AIDS-related Kaposi's sarcoma. Eur J Cancer Clin Oncol 1989 (25): 759-761

32 Spirtos NM, Smith LH and Teng NM: Prospective randomised trial of topical alpha-interferon (alpha-interferon gels) for the treatment of vulvar intraepithelial neoplasia III. Gynecol Oncol 1990 (37): 34-38

33 Rosso R, Rimoldi R, Salvatti F, De Palma M, Cinquegrana A, Nicolò G, Ardizzoni A, Fusco U, Cappaccio A, Centofanti R, Neri M, Cruciani AR and Maisto L: Intrapleural natural beta interferon in the treatment of malignant pleural effusions. Oncology 1988 (45): 253-256

34 Berek JS, Hacker, NF, Lichenstein A , Jung T, Spina C, Knox, RM, Brady J, Greene T, Ettinger LM and Lagasse LD: Intraperitoneal recombinant alpha-Interferon for salvage immunotherapy in stage III epithelial ovarian cancer. A Gynecologic Oncology Group study. Cancer Res 1985 (45): 4447-4453

35 Welander CE: Interferon in the treatment of ovarian cancer. Sem Oncol 1988 (15, suppl. 5): 26-29

36 Pujade-Lauraine E, Colombo N, Namer N, Fumoleau P, Monnier A, Nooy MA, Falkson G, Mignot L, Bugat R, Oliveira CMD, Mousseau M, Netter ZG, Oberling F, Coiffier B and Brandley M: Intraperitoneal human rIFN gamma in patients with residual ovarian carcinoma at second look laparotomy. Proc Am Soc Clin Oncol 1990 (9): 156

37 Lum BL and Torti FM: Therapeutic approaches including interferon to carcinoma in situ of the bladder. Cancer Treat Rev 1985 (12, suppl B): 45-59

38 Ackerman, D, Biedermann C, Bailly G, Studer UE: Treatment of superficial bladder tumour with intravesical recombinant interferon-α2a. Urol Int 1988 (43): 85-88

39 Chodak GW: Intravesical interferon treatment of superficial bladder cancer. Urology 1989 (34, suppl 4): 84-86

40 Kinnula V, Cantell K and Mattson K: Effect of inhaled natural interferon-alpha on diffuse bronchioalveolar carcinoma. Eur J Cancer 1990 (26): 740-741

41 van Zandwijk N, Jassem E, Dubbelmann R, Braat MCP and Rumke P: Aerosol application of interferon-alpha in the treatment of bronchioalveolar carcinoma. Eur J Cancer 1990 (26): 738-740

42 Rosenberg SA, Lotze MT, Yang JC, Linehan WM, Seipp, C, Calabro S, Karp SE, Sherry RM, Stenberg S and White DE: Combination therapy with interleukin-2 and alfa interferon for the treatment of patients with advanced cancer. J Clin Oncol 1989 (7): 1863-1874

43 Atzpodien J, Korfer A, Franks CR, Poliwoda H and Kirchner H: Home therapy with recombinant interleukin 2 and interferon α-2b in advanced human malignancies. Lancet 1990 (335): 1509-1512

44 Wadler S and Schwartz EL: Antineoplastic activity of the combination of interferon and cytotoxic agents against experimental and human malignancies: a review. Cancer Res 1990 (50): 3473-3486

45 Wadler S, Schwartz EL, Goldman M, Lyver A, Rader M, Zimmerman M, Itri L, Weinberg V and Wiernik PH: Fluorouracil and recombinant alpha-2a-interferon: an active regimen against advanced colorectal carcinoma. J Clin Oncol 1988 (7): 1769-1775

46 Wadler S and Wiernik PH: Clinical update on the role of fluorouracil and recombinant interferon alpha-2b in the treatment of colorectal carcinoma. Sem Oncol 1990 (17, suppl 1): 16-21

47 Balkwill FR: Peptide regulatory factors. Interferons. Lancet 1989 (1): 1060-1063

Interferons: Biosynthesis, Physiological Roles, Mechanisms of Induction and Response

George R. Stark

Imperial Cancer Research Fund, Lincoln's Inn Fields, London WC2A 3PX, United Kingdom

Interferons (IFNs) are members of the cytokine family of extracellular signalling proteins. There are 2 major types: alpha and beta IFNs (type I) act primarily to mediate resistance to viruses and as negative regulators of cell growth, whereas gamma IFN (type II) acts primarily to modulate immune responses within a complex network of other cytokines. However, the actions of the 2 types are not tightly confined, so that gamma IFN does have significant antiviral activity and alpha IFN has some role in immune modulation. Type I and type II IFNs have little homology and act through different cell surface receptors. However, recent work (see below) has revealed that there are common components in the signalling pathways through which the 2 types of IFN mediate their effects. For a recent general review of the IFNs, see Pestka et al. [1] and for a comprehensive review of the role of IFN in treating human neoplasia, with several sections of background information, see Strander [2].

Biosynthesis

This subject is well reviewed by Pestka et al. [1]. In man, there are at least 23 different alpha IFN genes, most of which are expressed, and single genes for beta and gamma IFNs, located on chromosomes 9, 9 and 12, respectively. Expression of the IFN genes is controlled with respect both to cell type and to the nature of the inducing stimulus. In general, alpha and gamma IFNs are induced more efficiently in peripheral blood cells and beta IFN is induced mainly in fibroblasts and epithelial cells. RNA viruses and double-stranded RNAs are efficient inducers of beta IFN in non-haemopoietic cells, whereas haemopoietic cells can express both alpha and beta IFN genes, but at different levels depending on the inducer and the cell type. It is interesting that other types of inducers, such as DNA viruses, several species of bacteria, or cells infected by DNA viruses can induce high levels of alpha IFN in a small but distinct population of peripheral blood lymphocytes [3]. In keeping with its primary role in mediating immune responses, gamma IFN is induced by antigens and mitogens in cells of the immune system. Other cytokines, such as tumour necrosis factors, colony stimulating factors and interleukins 1 and 2, can also induce the IFNs [4].

Physiological Roles

Rough extrapolations from the number of induced proteins seen in 2-dimensional gels or induced mRNAs represented in cDNA libraries indicate that 100 genes or more can respond to the IFNs. The nature of the response depends, as expected, on the cell type and the type of IFN used. Some genes respond in only one cell type; for example, complement factor B is induced only in endothelial cells [5]. Other genes respond predominantly to a single type of IFN in most cells, for example, the class II HLA genes to gamma IFN [1] and the human 6-16 gene to type I IFNs [6]. Alternatively, many genes respond to both types of IFN, for example the class I HLA genes [1] and the human 9-27 gene [7].

Antiviral Responses

The problem of controlling infection by many different types of virus is complex and it is likely that many IFN-induced proteins are assigned to this task. An IFN-producing animal needs to take account not only of the different life styles of different viruses but also of the need to inhibit the growth of each virus in several different ways, to minimise the chance that resistant viruses will evolve. With the exception of retroviruses, all RNA viruses carry a double-stranded RNA (dsRNA) genome or replicate their single-stranded RNA genomes through a dsRNA intermediate. Thus it is not surprising that the presence of dsRNA per se has been used as a cue to indicate infection by many different classes of viruses. dsRNA, released from virus-infected cells in a lytic infection or provided exogenously as poly(rI). poly(rC), is a potent inducer of beta IFN, and study of 2 different IFN-induced enzymes that are activated by dsRNA provides us with the best understood examples of antiviral mechanisms [8]. A dsRNA-activated protein kinase phosphorylates the translational initiation factor eIF-2, blocking its function and thus inhibiting protein synthesis in virus-infected cells but not in uninfected cells.

Another dsRNA-activated enzyme synthesises 2',5'-oligoadenylates from ATP, and these unusual molecules in turn activate a latent ribonuclease that destroys mRNAs and viral replicative intermediates in infected cells. As examples of other antiviral mechanisms, we know that the packaging of retroviruses into infectious particles is inhibited in IFN-treated cells and that a very early step in infection by the double-stranded DNA virus SV40 is blocked by IFN [9], but we have little idea of the mechanisms involved. Also, the IFN-induced protein Mx profoundly inhibits the growth of influenza viruses by mechanisms that are still largely unknown [10].

Viruses Fight Back I

Our antiviral mechanisms have co-evolved with the viruses, which have worked out ways to evade them. As one example, adenoviruses and Epstein-Barr virus encode small RNAs called VA and EBER, respectively, that are produced abundantly late in infection. These single-stranded RNAs have extensive self-complementarity and so fold back to a largely double-stranded structure. They bind to the IFN-induced protein kinase without activating it to phosphorylate eIF-2 and thus block this antiviral mechanism [11]. Poxviruses such as vaccinia achieve the same result through a viral protein that inhibits the same kinase. The poxviruses also inhibit activation of the latent ribonuclease by 2',5'-oligoadenylates [11].

Modulation of MHC Expression

A major function of the MHC gene products is to assist in presenting cell-associated antigens to T cells of the immune system. See Harding and Unanue [12] for a recent review. The antigens appear at the cell surface as peptides derived from partially degraded proteins, tightly bound to class I or class II MHC proteins. Many cells have low levels of MHC proteins but these levels increase substantially in response to alpha and gamma IFNs (class I MHC genes) or in response to gamma IFN (class II genes).

Role in Viral Infections

The class I MHC proteins bring peptides derived from intracellular antigens to the cell surface, where the complex stimulates a response from cytotoxic T cells. This mechanism provides a way to rid the body of cells expressing any protein to which the animal is not tolerant. For example, cells that do not display intact viral proteins on their surface can nevertheless be recognised and destroyed on the basis of internal viral proteins. The class II MHC proteins have a different function. They bring peptides derived from extracellular antigens (such as free virus particles) to the cell surface, where the complex stimulates responses from helper T cells. These function to facilitate both the humoural immune responses of B cells and the immune regulatory responses of cytotoxic T cells, which are thus stimulated to release a battery of cytokines. The cytokines in turn regulate the functions of many other cell types such as, for example, macrophages.

Thus, the pathway mediated by class II MHC proteins leads to production of large amounts of circulating antibody, appropriate for eliminating extracellular components, and to stimulation of cellular immune responses as well.

Viruses Fight Back II

Hepatocytes have very low levels of class I expression in the absence of induction but respond well to alpha, beta and gamma IFNs. Recent work [13] has indicated that the hepatitis B virus terminal protein, a subregion of the complex viral polymerase, can block the ability of cells to respond to both types of IFN. This activity blocks their ability to induce class I MHC expression and thus to present peptides derived from intracellular hepatitis B viral proteins. By this mechanism, some hepatocytes persistently infected by the hepatitis B virus evade destruction by cytotoxic T cells, helping to establish a long-term chronic infection resistant to endogenous or therapeutically administered IFN. Patients with IFN-resistant chronic infections eventually die from destruction of the liver caused by the virus, or from hepatocellular carcinoma. As an added factor, the same hepatitis B terminal protein also prevents cells from producing IFN in response to dsRNA.

A related story has been found for the E1A protein of adenovirus 5, which also seems able to block cellular responses to gamma IFN, alpha IFN and dsRNA. However, the hepatitis B and adenovirus proteins have no substantial homology and appear to block the response to alpha IFN at different points (Andrew M. Ackrill, Graham R. Foster, George R. Stark and Ian M. Kerr, unpublished). Tumour cells that fail to express MHC proteins may also fail to present viral or non-viral tumour antigens at the cell surface. If antigen presentation plays a role in recognition and destruction of cells by the immune system, loss of responsiveness of tumour cells to endogenous or therapeutically administered IFN could be a factor in allowing them to survive.

Antigrowth Responses

Much of the background information in this area has been reviewed by Strander [2]. Inhibition of cell growth *in vitro* by IFNs depends quite strongly on the type of cell and on the conditions. Low concentrations of IFN sufficient to induce a maximum antiviral response often do not inhibit cell growth, but high concentrations are sometimes effective. Cells respond to the combination of negative growth regulators, such as the IFNs, and positive regulators such as growth factors. In defined media, cells require more IFN to exhibit a given level of growth inhibition as the concentration of growth factors is increased [14]. In comparison with our understanding of the molecular bases of the antiviral effects of IFNs, where at least the tip of an iceberg is visible, we know virtually nothing about how growth inhibitory effects are mediated.

The antigrowth activity of the IFNs has obvious relevance to their antitumour activity, but interpretations of *in vivo* experiments are inevitably complicated by the multiple activities of the IFNs. Some of the complexity is revealed in experiments involving xenografts of human tumours transplanted into athymic (nude) mice [15]. Since IFNs are species specific, effects of human IFNs in this system are likely to be due to direct inhibition of growth of the tumour cells, whereas effects of mouse IFNs are probably due to activation of mouse inhibitory pathways. Consistent antitumour effects of human IFNs have been seen for renal, breast, ovarian and colorectal tumours and in osteosarcomas transplanted into nude mice. However, murine IFNs can also have antitumour effects against human xenografts in nude mice. Direct growth inhibition and activation of T cells is ruled out here, leaving some unknown modulation of the host-tumour interaction responsible for the growth inhibition observed.

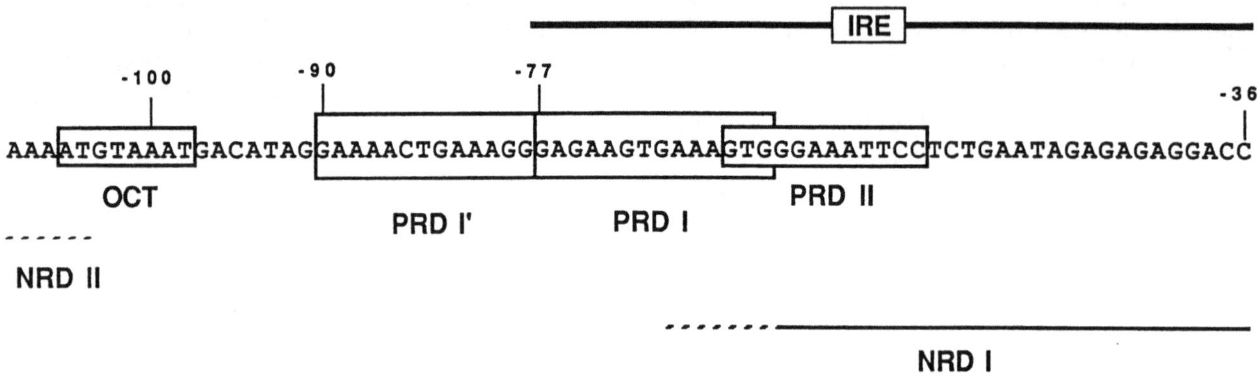

Fig. 1. Regulatory elements within the human beta-interferon promoter. Positive elements important for induction by double-stranded RNA or viral infection are boxed (OCT, PRDI', PRDI, PRDII). Note the similarity between PRDI [GAGAAGTGAAAGT] and the consensus ISRE of IFN-regulated genes [GGAAAN(N)GAAACT]. Negative regulatory domains (NRDI and II) are indicated by broken lines to show that they are dispersed and incompletely defined. IRE is the sequence sufficient to confer inducibility to a heterologous promoter. Nucleotide positions are relative to the start of transcription. This diagram is taken from Goodbourn [17].

Signalling Pathways for Production of the IFNs

Most of the work has been done with the human beta and alpha IFN genes [16,17]. Regulatory regions of DNA about 100 basepairs long lie immediately outside the sites where transcription of the IFN mRNAs begins (Fig. 1). These regions are quite complex, containing binding sites for several proteins that regulate transcription in different ways. There are sites for general transcription factors that participate in expression of many genes, for negative regulatory factors that help to keep the IFN genes turned off in the absence of an inducing signal, and for positive regulatory factors that are activated by signals provided by the introduction of dsRNA or viral particles into cells. Several of the proteins that bind to these regulatory sites have been defined and their roles are becoming understood. Nevertheless, despite years of effort by outstanding laboratories, we still do not know how cells sense the presence of the inducer and transmit the signals leading to removal of the inhibitory proteins and binding of the stimulatory proteins. Our best information is for induction by dsRNA, which may signal by activating a kinase similar or identical to the one that phosphorylates eIF-2 (see above). A possible substrate for this kinase would be an inactive transcription factor which becomes activated when phosphorylated. A candidate is the factor IRF-1, which seems to function both in inducing the IFNs and in responding to them (see below). It is possible that viruses can also trigger the production of IFNs through mechanisms that do not involve dsRNA, but the situation is not clear at present.

Response to Type I (alpha, beta) IFNs

We have come to know quite a lot about this pathway in the last few years. For a recent review, see Levy and Darnell [18].

Receptors

There are only a few thousand receptors per cell for type I IFNs, a low number compared to receptors for most other cytokines. Furthermore, a signal sufficient to activate expression of a hundred or more genes is generated when only a few IFN molecules are bound to the receptors of a single cell, so there must be amplification in the signalling pathway. The receptor is likely to be a complex protein composed of more than one subunit, by analogy to the more abundant receptors for other cytokines, characterised earlier, and from study of the properties of the subunit that binds IFNs. The gene encoding this subunit has recently been cloned [19], facilitating characterisation of the complete receptor.

There are interesting questions concerning the multiplicity of responses to type I IFNs. There is likely to be only one gene encoding the IFN-binding subunit, as judged by probing Southern transfers of genomic DNA with the cloned cDNA at high stringency. Yet there is a plethora of phenomena suggesting that the response is heterogeneous. For example, see the discussion on p.739 of Pestka et al. [1] describing quite different biological effects of different pure alpha IFN subtypes. In a similar vein, a mutant cell line that lacks any detectable response to alpha IFNs still retains a response to beta IFN [20]. Results such as these are difficult to reconcile with the simple model of a single receptor that recognises all type I IFNs and generates a single intracellular signal.

Signalling Pathways

It seems clear that several well studied "second messenger" pathways such as those involving the cyclic AMP-dependent kinase, protein kinase C or fluxes in intracellular pH or calcium concentration are not responsible for carrying the primary signal generated by binding of IFN to its receptor. Recent work of Hannigan and Williams [21] has, however, suggested a possible role for the phospholipase A_2-catalysed hydrolysis of arachidonic acid.

The pathway used by type I IFNs involves a mechanism quite different from those noted above. A specific intracellular protein transmits the signal from the cell surface to the DNA. The main features of the pathway are shown in Figure 2. Briefly, binding of IFN to its receptor leads to rapid conversion of a latent, inactive transcription factor to its active, DNA-binding form. The latent factor is present in the cytosol, possibly in close proximity to the receptor [22,23]. Upon activation, it moves rapidly to the nucleus, where it binds to the regulatory DNA elements that lie near the transcription start sites of the IFN-stimulated genes. These IFN-stimulated regulatory elements (ISREs) are highly conserved, conforming closely to the consensus sequence GGAAAN(N)GAAACT, where N is any nucleotide. The latent transcription factor, called E (or ISGF3), is composed of several subunits, and assembly of the complete active factor apparently takes place in the cytosol after activation. The entire process is very rapid: increased transcription is readily observed 1 minute after adding IFN to cells. We know most about the later events in this pathway, and very little about the nature of the signal that passes from the receptors to latent E factor. It seems probable that protein phosphorylation will be involved and that signal amplification takes place at this point.

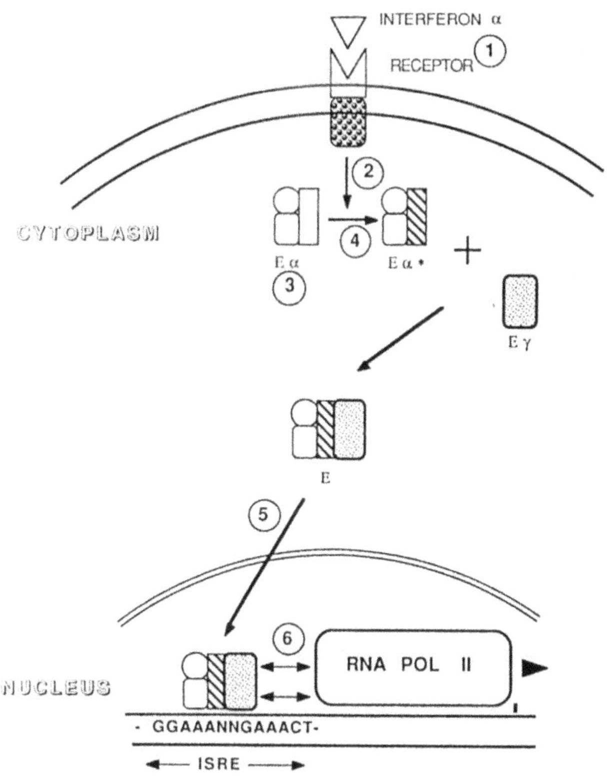

Fig. 2. Mechanisms of gene activation by alpha IFN. Some major features that are not well understood are, as numbered in the diagram: 1) The structure of the receptor, even though the subunit that binds alpha IFN has been cloned; 2) The nature of the first signal and the number of steps before activation of E alpha; 3) The subunit structure of E alpha. Possibly composed of 3 different polypeptides; 4) The nature of the modification responsible for activating E alpha to E alpha*, and why this permits association with E gamma; 5) How E is activated for transport to the nucleus; 6) How E interacts with components required for transcription.

Phospholipase A_2 may, for example, play a role in maintaining one or more of these early signalling proteins in an active state.
Once the IFN-regulated genes have been activated by the primary signal just described, secondary events determine the full time course of the response. These secondary events depend upon the properties of proteins whose synthesis is stimulated by the primary response. The level of active E factor declines within an hour or 2 after the cells have been treated with IFN. A second positively-acting factor called M (or ISGF2) then takes over, binding to the ISREs and maintaining transcription [24]. In time (usually 10-15 hours) the response is lost, even in the continued presence of IFN. Down-regulation probably involves several different processes including internalisation of occupied receptors (to stop them from generating any more signals), down-regulation of unoccupied receptors, disappearance of the positive transcription factors E and M, and possibly synthesis of negative factors that inhibit the signalling pathway. By means such as these the response to IFN is highly regulated both with respect to the levels of the IFN-induced proteins achieved and with respect to the length of time the cell is kept in the IFN-induced "on guard" state.

Response to Type II (gamma) IFN

The gamma IFN receptor is distinct from the alpha, beta receptor and there are about 10 times more gamma IFN receptors per cell. This relative abundance facilitated the earlier cloning of a cDNA encoding the IFN-binding subunit of the gamma receptor [25]. Genetic studies have made it clear that the gene for the IFN-binding subunit is on chromosome 6 and have also revealed a role for one or more genes on chromosome 21, probably encoding one or more additional subunits of a complex receptor.
In contrast to the situation for type I IFNs, the nature of the primary signal for response to gamma IFN is not yet well defined, although preliminary work has indicated that one or more transcription factors analogous to E in mode of activation (but clearly not E itself) are likely to be involved [18]. Since the primary transcription factor has not yet been defined, it is difficult to specify the sequence of gamma IFN ISREs in detail. By analogy to the "keep-on" factor M, a very similar positively acting factor called G is induced as part of the secondary response to gamma IFN [24]. M and G apparently include as one component IRF-1 [26], noted above and discussed again below, but these 2 factors may be be more complex and their composition and structure is not yet understood fully.
Many genes are regulated by both type I and type II IFNs, and this is probably achieved through identical or similar, partially overlapping ISREs. In addition, the class II MHC genes are induced only in response to gamma IFN. Since class II genes do not have the ISRE sequences noted above, they must respond to a primary or secondary signal different from those mediated through these sequences. Although there are conserved sequence elements in the regulatory regions of class II genes that are required for function, none has yet been found to bind a gamma IFN-induced factor [27].

Cross Talk

There are several intriguing connections between the pathways mediating synthesis of IFNs and those mediating the responses to IFNs. This situation is not wholly unexpected since one can imagine that the IFN system, which responds indirectly to a viral infection, may well have evolved from a simpler primordial system in which the antiviral response was direct and did not involve intercellular signalling. It has been known for quite a while that dsRNA is an important element in signalling the presence of a virus to the IFN genes themselves, but only more recently has it been appreciated that dsRNA also signals some of the IFN-responsive genes directly, without the need for IFN. This has been demonstrated most clearly in variant cell lines that do not produce or respond to IFNs, but nevertheless do show strong induction of several genes through direct response to dsRNA [28].

Another connection involves the transcription factor IRF-1, originally identified through its binding to regulatory elements of the alpha and beta IFN genes. After a cDNA clone for IRF-1 had been obtained, it was found that expression of the IRF-1 gene was stimulated both by viruses and by the IFNs [29]. The IRF-1 protein seems to be a positive regulator of both IFN gene expression and expression of IFN-responsive genes, in the latter case as an important constituent of the previously mentioned factors M and G. IRF-1 binds to similar DNA elements in the ISREs and in the regulatory regions of the alpha and beta IFN genes (see PRD1 in Fig.1). A related factor, IRF-2, binds to very similar elements but is likely to be a negative rather than a positive regulator. It is significant in this regard that IRF-2 appears later after induction by viruses or IFN than IRF-1 [30]. Recently, expression of human IRF-1 cDNA in the B-cell lineage of transgenic mice was achieved by utilising regulatory elements for human heavy chain expression. In such mice, the B-cell population was severely and specifically depleted, underscoring the possible importance of the IFNs as negative regulators of cell growth during normal development [31].

Finally, from studies of cells carrying mutations in the IFN response pathways, it has become evident that, although the pathways mediating responses to the 2 types of IFN must carry distinct and different signals, some components of the 2 pathways are shared in common. In particular, a mutant cell line called U2, selected to be defective in responding to type I IFNs, is also partially defective in several aspects of its response to gamma IFN [32]. Another mutant cell line selected with alpha IFN, not yet as well characterised as U2, seems to have lost the response to gamma IFN completely (David Flavell, Joseph John, George R. Stark, Ian M. Kerr, unpublished).

Future Work on Signalling Pathways

Biochemical Approaches

At the moment, the only components of the signalling pathway for response to alpha, beta IFNs that have been cloned are cDNAs encoding IRF-1 and the IFN-binding subunit of the receptor. Purification of E (ISGF3) has proceeded well and the availability of the several components of this oligomeric transcription factor should lead soon to cDNA clones and antibodies [33]. These key reagents will then make possible further study of the unknown early events in the pathway. As already noted, much more work needs to be done to bring the comparable early events for response to gamma IFN to the same state of knowledge. For both pathways, purification and cloning should eventually yield antibodies and cDNAs for the unknown components of the oligomeric type I and type II receptors, facilitating a detailed description of their modes of action. For induction of the IFNs, the primary mechanism of response to dsRNA still remains to be elucidated.

Genetic Approaches

A system has been set up to allow selection of cell lines defective in their response to alpha, beta IFNs, and several different mutant cell lines have been obtained so far [20,32]. Human HT1080 cells containing the E.coli guanine phosphoribosyl transferase (gpt) gene under the control of an ISRE express gpt under IFN control. There are good selection procedures using cytotoxic drugs both for and against expression of gpt so that, after treatment with a mutagen, cell lines defective in their response to IFN can be obtained. Such cell lines can then be transfected with genomic or cDNAs, followed by selection for restoration of IFN-induced gpt expression, to recover the wild-type version of the mutated genes. This approach should facilitate identification and isolation of components of the pathway that may be very difficult to obtain biochemically. For example, it is a major problem to purify a rare protein kinase whose substrate is unknown.

An alternative approach to selection with cytotoxic drugs is to isolate physically cells that have expressed a particular cell surface antigen in response to IFN, using specific antibodies and the fluorescence-activated cell sorter as tools. The antigens can be either endogenous proteins such as the class I and class II HLAs or the products of exogenous genes placed under control of ISREs and then transfected into cells. Complementation of mutant cell lines should provide cloned cDNAs and antibodies corresponding to crucial components of the signalling pathways. Also, when genetic manipulation of the cloned genes becomes possible, such cell lines can provide the null background in which different variant proteins can be tested, to facilitate fine definition of the properties and interactions of each signalling element.

REFERENCES

1 Pestka S, Langer JA, Zoon KC and Samuel CE: Interferons and their actions. Ann Rev Biochem 1987 (56):727-777

2 Strander H: Interferon treatment of human neoplasia. Advances Cancer Res 1986 (46)

3 Sandberg K, Matsson P and Alm GV: A distinct population of nonphagocytic and low level CD4+ null lymphocytes produce IFN-alpha after stimulation by herpes simplex virus-infected cells. J Immunol 1990 (145):1015-1020

4 Balkwill FR: Interferons. Lancet 1989 (i):1060-1063

5 Wu LC, Morley BJ and Campbell RD: Cell-specific expression of the human complement protein factor B gene: Evidence for the role of two distinct 5'-flanking elements. Cell 1987 (48):331-342

6 Kelly JM, Porter ACG, Chernajovsky Y, Gilbert CS, Stark GR and Kerr IM: Characterization of a human gene inducible by alpha- and beta-interferons and its expression in mouse cells. EMBO J 1986 (5):1601-1606

7 Reid LE, Brasnett AH, Gilbert CS, Porter ACG, Gewert DR, Stark GR and Kerr IM: A single DNA response element can confer inducibility by both alpha- and gamma-interferons. Proc Natl Acad Sci USA 1989 (86):840-844

8 Lengyel P: Biochemistry of interferons and their actions. Ann Rev Biochem 1982 (51):251-282

9 Brennan MB and Stark GR: Interferon pretreatment inhibits Simian virus 40 infections by blocking the onset of early transcription. Cell 1983 (33): 811-816

10 Aebi M, Fah J, Hurt N, Samuel CE, Thomis D, Bazzigher L, Pavlovic J, Haller O and Staeheli P: cDNA structures and regulation of two interferon-induced human Mx proteins. Mol Cell Biol 1989 (9): 5062-5072

11 Schneider RJ and Shenk T: Impact of virus infection on host cell protein synthesis. Ann Rev Biochem 1987 (56): 317-332

12 Harding CV and Unanue ER: Cellular mechanisms of antigen processing and the function of class I and II major histocompatibility complex molecules. Cell Reg 1990 (1):499-509

13 Foster GR, Ackrill AM, Goldin RD, Kerr IM, Thomas HC and Stark GR: Expression of the terminal protein region of hepatitis B virus inhibits cellular responses to alpha and gamma interferons and double-stranded RNA. Proc Natl Acad Sci USA 1991 (in press)

14 Taylor-Papadimitriou J, Shearer M and Rozengurt E: Inhibitory effect of interferon on cellular DNA synthesis: Modulation by pure mitogenic factors. J Interferon Res 1981 (1):401-409

15 Malik STA and Balkwill FR: The nude mouse in the study of cytokines. In: Boven E (ed) Nude Mouse in Cancer Research. Academic Press, Amsterdam (submitted)

16 Taniguchi T: Regulation of cytokine gene expression. Ann Rev Immunol 1988 (6):439-464

17 Goodbourn S: The regulation of beta-interferon gene expression. Seminars in Cancer Biology 1990 (1):89-95

18 Levy D and Darnell Jr JE: Interferon-dependent transcriptional activation: Signal transduction without second messenger involvement. The New Biologist 1990 (2):923-928

19 Uze G, Lutfalla G and Gresser I: Genetic transfer of a functional human interferon alpha receptor into mouse cells: Cloning and expression of its cDNA. Cell 1990 (60):225-234

20 Pellegrini S, John J, Shearer M, Kerr IM and Stark GR: Use of a selectable marker regulated by alpha interferon to obtain mutations in the signaling pathway. Mol Cell Biol 1989 (9):4605-4612

21 Hannigan GE and Williams BRG: Signal transduction by interferon-alpha through arachidonic acid metabolism. Science 1991 (251):204-207

22 Dale TC, Imam AMA, Kerr IM and Stark GR: Rapid activation by interferon alpha of a latent DNA-binding protein present in the cytoplasm of untreated cells. Proc Natl Acad Sci USA 1989 (86):1203-1207

23 Levy DE, Kessler DS, Pine R and Darnell Jr JE: Cytoplasmic activation of ISGF3, the positive regulator of interferon-alpha-stimulated transcription, reconstituted in vitro. Genes and Develop 1989 (3):1362-1371

24 Imam AMA, Ackrill AM, Dale TC, Kerr IM and Stark GR: Transcription factors induced by interferons

alpha and gamma. Nucl Acids Res 1990 (18): 6573-6580

25 Aguet M, Dembic Z and Merlin G: Molecular cloning and expression of the human interferon-gamma receptor. Cell 1988 (55): 273-280

26 Pine R, Decker T, Kessler DS, Levy DE and Darnell Jr JE: Purification and cloning of interferon-stimulated gene factor 2 (ISGF2): ISGF2 (IRF-1) can bind to the promoters of both beta interferon and interferon-stimulated genes but is not a primary transcriptional activator of either. Mol Cell Biol 1990 (10):2448-2457

27 Yang Z, Sugawara M, Ponath PD, Wessendorf L, Banerji J, Li Y and Strominger JL: Interferon gamma response region in the promoter of the human DPA gene. Proc Natl Acad Sci USA 1990 (87): 9226-9230

28 Wathelet MC, Clauss IM, Paillard FC and Huez GA: 2-aminopurine selectively blocks the transcriptional activation of cellular genes by virus, double-stranded RNA and interferons in human cells. Eur J Biochem 1989 (184):503-509

29 Taniguchi T: Regulation of interferon-beta gene: structure and function of cis-elements and trans-acting factors. J Interferon Res 1989 (9): 633-640

30 Harada H, Fujita T, Miyamoto M, Kimura Y, Maruyama M, Furia A, Miyata T and Taniguchi T: Structurally similar but functionally distinct factors, IRF-1 and IRF-2, bind to the same regulatory elements of IFN and IFN-inducible genes. Cell 1989 (58):729-739

31 Yamada G, Ogawa M, Akagi K, Miyamoto H, Nakano N, Itoh S, Miyazaki J-I, Nishikawa S-I, Yamamura K-I and Taniguchi T: Specific depletion of the B-cell population induced by aberrant expression of human interferon regulatory factor 1 gene in transgenic mice. Proc Natl Acad Sci USA 1991 (88):532-536

32 John J, McKendry R, Pellegrini S, Flavell D, Kerr IM and Stark GR: Isolation and characterisation of a new mutant human cell line unresponsive to alpha, beta interferon. Mol Cell Biol 1991 (submitted)

33 Fu X-Y, Kessler DS, Veals SA, Levy DE and Darnell Jr JE: ISGF3, the transcriptional activator induced by interferon alpha, consists of multiple interacting polypeptide chains. Proc Natl Acad Sci USA 1990 (87): 8555-8559

The Mechanisms of Action and the Role of Alpha Interferon in the Therapy of Myeloma

A. Österborg and H. Mellstedt, for the Myeloma Group of Central Sweden (MGCS)

Department of Oncology (Radiumhemmet), Karolinska Hospital, S-104 01 Stockholm, Sweden

Intermittent high-dose melphalan/prednisone (MP) treatment [1] is regarded by many clinicians as first-line therapy for patients with multiple myeloma. The introduction of intensive combination chemotherapy has not been shown to consistently improve the response rate or to prolong survival [2,3]. Since the overall prognosis for myeloma patients is rather poor, there is a need for better treatment modalities.

Alpha-interferon (alpha-IFN) is a biological therapeutic which has demonstrated antitumoural effects in various experimental systems and in humans [4-7]. Among haematological malignancies, hairy cell leukaemia and chronic granulocytic leukaemia show an excellent response to alpha-IFN [8,9]. Both natural and recombinant alpha-IFN have documented effects.

Mechanisms of Action of IFN

The exact mechanisms for the antitumoural activities of alpha-IFN are still unknown. It can be assumed that several functions might be operating. A summary of possible mechanisms in myeloma is shown in Table 1.

A direct cytotoxic effect of alpha-IFN on cultured myeloma plasma cells has been observed [10,11]. In some cases, selective down-regulation of the monoclonal immunglobulin production without a decrease in myeloma cell viability has also been noted [12]. A dose-dependent growth-inhibitory effect of interferon has been described in several experimental systems including myeloma [13,14]. It is controversial whether such a relationship exists *in vivo* [15], although there are clinical observations which might indicate that such a correlation may exist [16].

The cytotoxic effect of alpha-IFN might be enhanced when combined with chemotherapeutic agents. In an *in vitro* colony-formation assay, an additive cytotoxic effect was seen when IFN was combined with prednisone. IFN in combination with melphalan resulted in a synergistic growth inhibitory effect. When all 3 agents were added together an even greater cytotoxic activity was noted [17]. This study showed also a dose-dependent effect of alpha-IFN.

IFN might influence the pharmacokinetics of melphalan. A decrease in AUC (area under the concentration curve) of melphalan was observed when administered together with alpha-IFN [18]. This effect might be ascribed to IFN itself, or to the elevated body temperature induced by IFN. The clinical significance of the finding is not yet established, but might indicate an increased cellular uptake of melphalan with a concomitant increase in the cytotoxic effect.

IFN has been shown to inhibit the growth-promoting effect of various growth factors. Cell lines dependent on epidermal growth factor (EGF) or platelet-derived growth factor (PDGF) for proliferation *in vitro* were arrested after addition of IFN, probably by interference with the binding of the growth factors to the cell surface receptors [19]. In hairy cell leukaemia IFN has been found to inhibit the growth-promoting effect of low molecular BCGF [20]. Maybe a similar inhibitory effect of IFN on IL-6 induced myeloma cell growth might be operating. This assumption fits in

Table 1. Tentative mechanisms of action of alpha-IFN *in vivo* in the treatment of multiple myeloma

Function	Ref
A direct cytotoxic effect	10, 11
A synergistic cytotoxic effect with alkylating agents and prednisone	17
A decrease of monoclonal immunoglobulin production without affecting myeloma cell viability	12
A change in the pharmacokinetics of melphalan	18
Inhibition of growth promoting effect of various growth factors	19, 20
Down-regulation of oncogene expression	22
Increase in NK cell functions	27
Increase in the tumour cell surface antigens and augmentation of immunogenicity	30
Expansion of specific T-cells	29
Induction of differentiation of malignant progenitor cells	31

well with some clinical observations. A high responsiveness to IL-6 was found in myeloma cells from patients with stage I disease compared to stage III myeloma [21]. Patients with a low tumour burden showed a significantly higher anti-tumour response to IFN than patients with advanced disease (see below).

Another IFN-mediated effect might be down-regulation of oncogenes. IFN has been shown to down-regulate various oncogenes in experimental systems [22]. Amplification of the c-myc and bcl-1 oncogenes and ras mutation has been described in myeloma [23,24] as well as various chromosomal translocations [25]. Thus, IFN might also inhibit myeloma tumour cell progression by down-regulation of oncogenes.

In vitro and *in vivo* natural killer (NK) cell activity may be enhanced by IFN. An increase in NK cell functions has been described in myeloma patients with a low tumour burden and in patients responding to therapy, while patients with advanced disease had an impaired NK activity [26]. Thus, patients with a low tumour mass seem to have an intact NK cell system which may be functionally augmented after IFN administration [27] and thereby exert antitumoural effects.

In a mouse myeloma system, idiotype-reactive T cells with specific inhibitory functions on the expanding myeloma clone have been described [28]. Idiotype-reactive T cells have been found also in human myeloma (data to be published). IFN can enhance a specific T cell response [29] and thus IFN-stimulated expansion of specific T cells might also be a possible mechanism of action as well as increased immunogenicity of the tumour cells by increased expression of MHC and tumour-associated antigens [30].

IFN induces differentiation of chronic lymphocytic leukaemia cells [31] which might lead to tumour cell death. A similar mechanism may be operating in the precursor B lymphocyte pool of the myeloma tumour cell clone [32], as the major proliferative activity in multiple myeloma seems to be confined to the precursor B cell compartment [33,34].

In summary, various direct or indirect IFN-mediated effects might be operating to explain the antitumoural effects in multiple myeloma. These findings may have therapeutic implications. It is suggested that at diagnosis, when the tumour cell compartment is large and the proliferating capacity comparatively high, IFN should be combined with chemotherapy in order to utilise a direct cytotoxic effect and to obtain maximal tumour reduction within a short time. In the response/plateau phase, which is characterised by a low proliferative capacity of the myeloma cells, IFN may be used alone or in combination with other cytokines to await the effects on various immune functions.

Induction Therapy with Interferon. Results of MGCS Studies

Since 1976, the Myeloma Group of Central Sweden (MGCS) has studied the therapeutic effect of natural alpha-IFN in previously untreated patients with multiple myeloma. In a randomised trial, a dose of 3 x 10^6 U of alpha-IFN daily was compared to MP. The response rate in IgG myelomas was low (5%) while in IgA and Bence-Jones (BJ) myelomas the response frequency (26%) was not statistically different from that of MP-treated patients [35]. This IFN dose was well tolerated without adverse side-effects. The overall survival did not differ significantly between the 2 treatment groups.

To meet the dose-dependent concept, 50 patients with IgA and Bence-Jones myelomas entered a pilot study using high doses of natural alpha-IFN [16]. This study showed that the highest dose tested, 30 x 10^6 U of alpha-IFN daily, caused unacceptable adverse reactions. The maximal tolerable dose that could be given with only minor side-effects to most patients was 10 x 10^6 U daily for 7 consecutive days repeated every third week. The overall response rate was 36%. The highest response frequencies were seen in those treatment groups that received the highest IFN dose, which, however, was associated with unacceptable toxicity. Response duration was usually of considerable length, exceeding 1 year in 11 out of 18 responding patients. The median survival was more than 3 years.

The results of these studies clearly demonstrated the beneficial effect of alpha-IFN as a single agent for induction therapy in multiple myeloma, although the clinical effect was not superior to conventional chemotherapy with regard to response frequency, response duration and survival.

Based on these results and on *in vitro* studies showing a synergistic growth inhibitory effect between interferon, melphalan and prednisone [17], a randomised study was initiated in April 1986. The patients were allotted to either intermittent melphalan (0.25 mg/kg/day)/ prednisone (2 mg/kg/day) for 4 consecutive days repeated every sixth week (MP) or to intermittent MP every sixth week plus 7 x 10^6 U/m^2/day of alpha-IFN for 5 consecutive days repeated every third week. When the patient obtained a response, MP was continued but the IFN dose was reduced to 3 x 10^6 U/day 3 days a week continuously (MP/IFN). Treatment was continued to progression or relapse. At progression/relapse all patients received the same combination chemotherapy regimen.

An interim analysis was performed in December 1990 [36]. Pretreatment characteristics of the patients are shown in Table 2.

The response frequencies are shown in Table 3. A statistically significant higher response rate was noted in the MP/IFN group compared to those receiving MP therapy only. In clinical stage II the response rate was significantly higher in the MP/IFN group than in the MP group while in stage III the difference between the 2 groups was not statistically significant. Patients with IgA or Bence-Jones myelomas showed a significantly higher response rate in the MP/IFN group than in the MP group, while in IgG myelomas the response frequency was numerically higher in the MP/IFN group although the difference was not statistically significant.

Sixty percent of the patients had no reduction of the IFN dose during the induction period. In 19 patients (15%), IFN had to be withdrawn due to side-effects. The reasons for withdrawal were the following: 1 myocardial infarction, 1 congestive heart failure, 1 coma with hemiparesis, 5 flu-like syndrome, 1 mental confusion, 2 allergic reaction, 1 throm-

Table 2. Pretreatment characteristics of the patients

	MP group	MP/IFN group
Total number of patients	154	146
Clinical		
stage II	68	62
stage III	86	84
S-creatinine		
<170 mmol/l	120	113
≥170 mmol/l	34	33
M-component		
IgG	81	78
IgA	36	33
Bence-Jones	30	30
Non-secretory	6	5
IgD	1	-
Number of patients evaluable for response (December 1990)	134	133

bocytopenia, 1 depressive symptoms, 2 renal dysfunction and 4 due to practical problems. In 25% of patients, various dose reductions were made. There were no major differences in haematological toxicity between the 2 treatment groups.

In the total material there was no difference in total survival between the 2 treatment groups. However, patients with IgA and Bence-Jones myeloma had a significant prolongation of total survival ($p<0.05$) in the MP/IFN treatment group.

The present study shows that MP/IFN therapy is an effective treatment for patients with multiple myeloma and superior to standard MP treatment with regard to response induction. The most pronounced effect was seen in patients with a low tumour mass (stage II) and in patients with IgA or Bence-Jones myeloma.

Induction Therapy with Interferon. Results of Other Studies

Several other reports have confirmed the therapeutic effect of alpha-IFN used as a single agent in the treatment of multiple myeloma [37]. IgA myelomas have also in some studies demonstrated a favourable response to IFN therapy [35,38,39]. The response frequencies of other studies comparing chemotherapy + IFN with chemotherapy alone are shown in Table 4.

Table 3. Response frequency (%) in relation to treatment schedule

	MP group (n=134)*	MP/IFN group (n=133)*	p-value
Total	45	65	<0.01
Clinical			
stage II	43 (26/60)	74 (43/58)	<0.01
stage III	46 (34/74)	57 (43/75)	n.s.
M-component			
IgG	51 (36/71)	59 (44/74)	n.s.
IgA	45 (15/33)	84 (26/31)	<0.01
Bence-Jones	30 (8/27)	62 (16/26)	<0.05

* Number of evaluable patients at analysis

n.s. = not significant

Table 4. Response frequencies (%) of alpha-IFN and chemotherapy for induction treatment of previously untreated multiple myeloma patients

Treatment schedule	Response rate (%) Mean	95% Confidence limits	Reference
MP (n=21)	71	(50-92)	Montuoro et al. [40]
MP/alpha-IFN (n=16)	81	(60-100)	
MP (n=24)	54	(33-75)	Corrado et al. [41]
MP/alpha-IFN (n=29)	41 (CR 7%)	(22-60)	
MP (n=134)	44	(35-54)	Cooper et al. [42]
MP/alpha-IFN (n=135)	37	(29-45)	
VBMCP/alpha-IFN (n=54)	80% (CR 26%)	(69-91)	Kyle et al. [43]
VMCP (n=27)	41	(22-60)	Ludvig et al. [44]
VMCP/alpha-IFN (n=21)	57	(34-80)	

CR = complete remission

A high response rate for MP/IFN (81%) was noted by Montuoro et al. [40]. In a study by Corrado et al. [41] no increase in the response frequency was seen for the MP/IFN combination although complete remissions, i.e., disappearance of the M-protein and normalisation of the bone marrow, were found in this group. Complete remission in multiple myeloma is a rare event. Cooper et al. [42] noted no increase in the response rate for an MP/IFN regimen (37%) compared to MP alone (44%). Response duration time as well as total survival were similar in both groups. However, the treatment regimens used by Corrado et al. and Cooper et al. were quite different from that of the MGCS trial both with regard to dose and scheduling. This indicates that it might be important how alpha-IFN is administered. Kyle et al. [43] reported in a non-randomised study that 80% of previously untreated patients responded to VBMCP + alpha-IFN and that 26% of the patients achieved a complete remission. Using a combination of VMCP and alpha-IFN compared to VMCP alone, Ludwig et al. [44] demonstrated superiority of the IFN-containing regimen for response induction, 57% vs. 41%.

Interferon as Maintenance Therapy

Another approach for alpha-IFN in multiple myeloma has been explored by the Italian Multiple Myeloma Study Group. After induction chemotherapy, responding patients were randomised to low-dose alpha-IFN (3 x 10^6 U/m^2 3 times a week) continuously or to no

Table 5. Response duration time and survival from response of multiple myeloma patients treated with or without alpha-IFN as maintenance therapy

Study group		Treatment groups	No. pts.	Response duration time (median) (months)	Survival from response (median) (months)
Italian Multiple Myeloma Study Group		No treatment	39	14	39
		vs		$p<0.001$	$p<0.01$
		α-IFN alone	38	32	51
Myeloma Group of Western Sweden		No treatment	53	6	No information
		vs		$p<0.01$	
		α-IFN alone	50	18	
MGCS	All pts	MP	60	20	23
		vs		NS	NS
		MP + α-IFN	86	29	31
	Stage II	MP	26	19	24
		vs		$p<0.01$	$p<0.001$
		MP + α-IFN	43	36	41
	Stage III	MP	34	20	21
		vs		NS	NS
		MP + α-IFN	43	15	18

NS = not significant

maintenance therapy [45]. The results of 3 studies using alpha-IFN as maintenance therapy are shown in Table 5.

A significantly longer response duration time and survival was found for patients receiving IFN therapy. A similar study is conducted by the Myeloma Group of Western Sweden [46]. Also in this study a significant prolongation of the response duration time was found.

The MGCS study differs from the 2 above-mentioned trials in that chemotherapy (MP) was continued during the response phase in both treatment groups. In the total patient material there was no difference in response duration time and survival from response. However, patients with a low tumour mass (stage II) receiving alpha-IFN had a statistically significant prolongation of response duration time ($p<0.01$) as well as survival from response ($p<0.001$).

There is now substantial evidence showing the superiority of chemotherapy in combination with alpha-IFN for response induction in myeloma as compared to chemotherapy alone. The results of the Italian Multiple Myeloma Study Group and of the present MGCS study support the notion that alpha-IFN may also have an impact on survival.

Acknowledgements

This study was supported by grants from the Swedish Cancer Society and the Cancer Society in Stockholm. For excellent secretarial help we thank Ms Marie Karlsson.

Members of MGCS:

M. Björkholm[2], M. Björeman[7], G. Brenning[6], K. Carlsson[6], G. Gahrton[5], G. Grimfors[2], H. Gyllenhammar[4], R. Hast[3], B. Johansson[1], G. Juliusson[5], M. Järnmark[7], A. Killander[6], E. Kimby[3], R. Lerner[4], H. Mellstedt[1] (chairman), K. Merk[1], M. Ohrling[5], C. Paul[5], B. Simonsson[6], B. Smedmyr[6], A.-M. Stalfelt[7], H. Strander[1], E. Svedmyr[1], A.-M. Udén[4], B. Wadman[7], E. Ösby[2], A. Österborg[1] (secretary).

The following departments participate in MGCS:

1) Department of Oncology (Radiumhemmet), 2) Department of Medicine, Karolinska Hospital, 3) Department of Medicine, Danderyds Hospital, 4) Department of Medicine, South Hospital, 5) Department of Medicine, Huddinge Hospital, Stockholm, 6) Department of Medicine, Academic Hospital, Uppsala, 7) Department of Medicine, Örebro Hospital, Sweden.

REFERENCES

1 Alexanian R, Haut A, Khan A et al: Treatment for multiple myeloma. Combination chemotherapy with different melphalan dose regimens. JAMA 1969 (208):1680-1685

2 Sporn JR and McIntyre OR: Chemotherapy of previously untreated multiple myeloma patients: An analysis of recent treatment results. Semin Oncol 1986 (13):318-325

3 Österborg A, Åhre A, Björkholm M et al: Alternating combination chemotherapy (VMCP/VBAP) is not superior to melphalan/prednisone in the treatment of multiple myeloma patients stage III - A randomized study from MGCS. Eur J Hematol 1989 (43):54-62

4 Taylor JL, Sabran JL and Grossberg SE: The cellular effects of interferon. In: Came PE, Carter WA (eds) Interferons and Their Applications. Springer-Verlag, New York 1984 pp 169-205

5 Weck PK and Came PE: Comparative biologic activities of human interferon. In: Came PE, Carter WA (eds) Interferons and Their Applications. Springer-Verlag, New York 1984 pp 339-357

6 Salmon SE and Ozer H: Alpha interferon therapy in oncology: Clinical update. Semin Oncol 1986 (13):1-2

7 Strander H: Interferon treament of human neoplasia. Adv Cancer Res 1986 (46):1-256

8 Ratain MJ, Vardiman JW and Golomb HM: The role of interferon in the treatment of hairy cell leukemia. Semin Oncol 1986 (13):21-28

9 Talpaz M, McCredie KB, Mavligit GM and Gutterman JU: Leukocyte interferon-induced myeloid cytoreduction in chronic myelogenous leukemia. Blood 1983 (62):689-692

10 Aapro MS, Alberts DS and Salmon SE: Interactions of human leukocyte interferon with vinca alkaloids and other chemotherapeutic agents against human tumors in clonogenic assay. Cancer Chemother Pharmacol 1983 (10):161-166

11 Einhorn S, Fernberg JO, Grandér D and Lewensohn R: Interferon exerts a cytotoxic effect on primary human myeloma cells. Eur J Cancer Clin Oncol 1988 (24):1505-1510

12 Grandér D, von Stedingk LV, Wasserman J and Einhorn S: Influence of interferon on antibody production and viability of malignant cells from patients with multiple myeloma. Eur J Haematol 1991 (46):17-25

13 Adams A, Strander H and Cantell K: Sensitivity of the Epstein-Barr virus transformed human lymphoid cell lines to interferon. J Gen Virol 1975 (28):207-217

14 Einhorn S and Strander H: Interferon therapy for neoplastic diseases in man: In vitro and in vivo studies. Adv Exp Med Biol 1978 (110):159-174

15 Case DC, Someborn HL, Paul SD et al: Phase II study of rDNA alpha-2 interferon (Intron A) in patients with multiple myeloma utilizing an escalating induction phase. Cancer Treat Rep 1986 (70):1251-1254

16 Åhre A, Björkholm M, Österborg A et al: High doses of natural alpha-interferon (α-IFN) in the treatment of multiple myeloma. - A pilot study from the Myeloma Group of Central Sweden (MGCS). Eur J Haematol 1988 (41):123-130

17 Cooper MR and Welander CE: Interferon in the treatment of multiple myeloma. Semin Oncol 1986 (13):334-340

18 Ehrsson H, Eksborg S, Wallin I, Österborg A and Mellstedt H: Oral melphalan pharmacokinetics - influence of interferon induced fever. Clin Pharmacother 1990 (47):86-90

19 Friedman RM: Growth factors, oncogenes, and interferon. J Exp Pathol 1986 (2):223-228

20 Paganelli KA, Evans SS, Han T and Ozer H: B cell growth factor-induced proliferation of hairy cell lymphocytes and inhibition by type 1 interferon in vitro. Blood 1986 (67):937-942

21 Asaoku H, Kawano M, Iwato K et al: Decrease in BSF-2/IL-6 response in advanced cases of multiple myeloma. Blood 1988 (2):429-432

22 Clemens M: Interferons and oncogenes. Nature 1985 (313):531-532

23 Pegoraro L, Malavesi F and Bellone G et al: The human myeloma cell line LP-1: A versatile model in which to study early plasma cell differentiation and c-myc activation. Blood 1989 (73):1020-1027

24 Krolewski JJ and Dalla-Favera R: Oncogenes and their relevance in the pathogenesis of hematologic malignancies. In: Luzzatto L, Mauer AM (eds) Education Book. Milan: XXII. Internat Congr of Hematol. 28 Aug - 3 Sept, 1988 pp 20-28

25 Gazdar AF, Oie HK, Kirsch IR and Hollis GF: Establishment and characterization of a human plasma cell myeloma culture having a rearranged cellular myc proto-oncogene. Blood 1986 (67):1542-1549

26 Österborg A, Nilsson B, Björkholm M, Holm G and Mellstedt H: Natural killer cell activity in monoclonal gammopathies: Relation to disease activity. Eur J Haematol 1990 (45):153-157

27 Einhorn S, Åhre A, Blomgren H et al: Interferon and natural killer activity in multiple myeloma. Lack of correlation between interferon induced enhancement of natural killer activity and clinical

response to human interferon-alpha. Int J Cancer 1982 (30): 167-172

28 Flood PM, Phillips C, Taupier MA and Schreiber H: Regulation of myeloma growth in vitro by idiotype-specific T lymphocytes. J Immunol 1980 (124):424-430

29 Lindahl P, Leary P and Gresser I: Enhancement by interferon of the specific cytotoxicity of sensitized lymphocytes. Proc Natl Acad Sci USA 1972 (69):1721-1725

30 Lindahl P, Gresser I, Leary P and Tovey M: Interferon treatment of mice: enhanced expression of histocompatibility antigens on lymphoid cells. Proc Natl Acad Sci USA 1976 (73):1284-1287

31 Tötterman TH, Danersund A, Carlsson M and Nilsson K: Effect of recombinant interferon-alpha and gamma on B-CLL cells in serum-free medium: Expression of activation, differentiation, and CALLA antigens. Leukemia 1987 (1):667-679

32 Mellstedt H, Holm G and Björkholm M: Multiple myeloma, Waldenström's macroglobulinemia and benign monoclonal gammopathy. Characteristics of the B cell clone, immunoregulatory cell populations and clinical implications. Adv Cancer Res 1984 (41): 257-289

33 Mellstedt H, Killander D and Pettersson D: Bone marrow kinetic studies on three patients with myelomatosis. Indications for malignant proliferation within both the plasma cell and lymphoid cell compartments. Acta Med Scand 1977 (202):413-417

34 Chan C, Wormsley SB, Pierce LE, Peter JB and Schechter GP: B-cell surface phenotypes of proliferating myeloma cells: Target antigens for immunotherapy. Am J Hematol 1989 (33):101-109

35 Åhre A, Bjrkholm M, Mellstedt H et al: Human leukocyte interferon and intermittent high dose melphalan/prednisolone administration in the treatment of multiple myeloma. A randomized clinical trial. Cancer Treat Rep 1984 (68):1331-1338

36 Mellstedt H, for the Myeloma Group of Central Sweden (MGCS): MP/alpha-IFN in the induction treatment of multiple myeloma and as maintenance therapy. - A randomized trial from MGCS. Abstract. IIIrd International Workshop on Multiple Myeloma, Torino, April 9-12, 1991

37 Österborg A and Mellstedt H: Induction therapy with interferon in multiple myeloma and possible mechanisms of action. In: Gutterman J, Talpaz M (eds) Biological Response Modifiers in Hematological Malignancies. Marcel Dekker Inc, New York 1990 (in press)

38 Ohno R and Kimura K: Treatment of multiple myeloma with recombinant interferon alfa-2a. Cancer 1986 (57):1685-1688

39 Ludwig H, Cortelezzi A, Scheithauer W et al: Recombinant interferon alfa-2C versus polychemotherapy (VMCP) for treatment of multiple myeloma: a prospective randomized trial. Eur J Cancer Clin Oncol 1986 (22):1111-1116

40 Montuoro A, De Rosa L and De Blasio A: Alpha-2-interferon/melphalan/prednisone versus melphalan/prednisone in previously untreated patients with multiple myeloma: Preliminary results. Abstract. XXII. Internat Congr of Hematol, 28 Aug - 3 Sept, Milan, Italy 1988

41 Corrado C, Pavlovsky S, Saslasky J et al: Randomized trial comparing melphalan-prednisone with or without recombinant alpha 2 interferon (r-alpha-2-IFN) in multiple myeloma. Proc Am Soc Clin Oncol (ASCO) 1989 (8):258 (abstr)

42 Cooper MD: Melphalan/Prednisone with and without alfa 2b interferon (IFN) in newly diagnosed multiple myeloma. 15th Int Cancer Congr, 16-22 Aug, Hamburg, Germany 1990, p 986 (abstract)

43 Kyle RA, Oken MM, Greipp PR, Kay NE and Tsiatis A: VBMCP/rIFN alpha 2 induction therapy in multiple myeloma. Vth Hannover Interferon Workshop, 21-23 February 1990, p 46 (abstr)

44 Ludwig J, Preis P, Scheithauer W et al: Interferon-alpha-2 (rIFN) with or without chemotherapy in newly-diagnosed patients with multiple myeloma. Proc Am Soc Clin Oncol (ASCO) 1989, A1080 (abstr)

45 Mandelli F, Avvisati G, Amadori S et al: Maintenance treatment with recombinant interferon alfa-2b in patients with multiple myeloma responding to conventional induction chemotherapy. N Engl J Med 1990 (20):1430-1434

46 Westin J, Cortelezzi A, Hjort M, et al: Interferon-alfa-2b therapy during the plateau phase of multiple myeloma. Vth Hannover Interferon Workshop 21-23 February 1990, p 50 (abstr)

The Role of Interferon in the Management of Low-Grade Lymphoma

Ama Rohatiner

ICRF Department of Medical Oncology, St. Bartholomew's Hospital, West Smithfield, London EC1A 7BE, U.K.

With the publication of Hans Strander's work on the use of interferon as adjuvant therapy following surgery for osteogenic sarcoma [1], attention focused on the potential role of interferon in the treatment of malignant disease. Disappointingly, it soon became clear that in the majority of common cancers, interferon is ineffectual. However, with regard to haematological malignancy, it was subsequently shown to be active in hairy-cell leukaemia [2-5], the myeloproliferative disorders chronic myeloid leukaemia [6,7] and essential thrombocythaemia [8], myeloma [9] and low-grade lymphoma [10-17].

During the last 10 years, interferons have been evaluated in a relatively small number of patients with lymphoma, but it has become apparent that whilst significant responses have been observed in patients with follicular lymphoma, interferons have little activity against intermediate and high-grade disease [10-12, 16-18]. The other area of interest has been cutaneous T-cell lymphoma. Some new (and old) data relating to both will be reviewed.

Follicular Lymphoma

Follicular lymphoma is an enigmatic disease: on the one hand, the majority of patients respond to treatment, be it chemotherapy or irradiation, indeed they may respond repeatedly, and yet the disease remains incurable, the inexorable pattern of relapse making death from lymphoma virtually inevitable. A new approach is therefore urgently needed.

Interferon as a Single Agent

The first studies in lymphoma used IFN-alpha obtained from 'buffy coats', at an empirical, relatively low dose, which had been shown to be consistent with a normal, ambulatory lifestyle, as determined in the Scandinavian osteogenic sarcoma studies [1]. In approximately one third of patients with follicular lymphoma in whom conventional therapy had failed, objective responses (usually partial) were observed and the side-effects were, in general, tolerable [10-16,18]. With the advent of recombinant DNA techniques, recombinant interferon preparations became available, making it possible to evaluate the drug on a more systematic basis. The more recent studies (in both previously treated and newly diagnosed patients) have confirmed the earlier results, with responses (again most frequently incomplete) being seen in approximately 50% of patients (Table 1).

Table 1. Response rates with recombinant and non-recombinant interferons

	CR+PR	No. pts.	Ref.
Non-recombinant IFNs			
IFN-α	3	6	[12]
IFN-α	4	8	[10]
IFN-α	3	18	[11]
Recombinant IFNs			
IFN-αA	6	17	[13]
IFN-αA *	4	9	[14]
IFN-αA	13	24	[18]
IFN-αA *	15	30	[16]
TOTAL	53	120	

* previously untreated patients

In a French study, when interferon was prospectively compared with prednimustine (a combination of prednisolone and chlorambucil) and an expectant policy, in newly diagnosed patients with follicular lymphoma deemed not to be in need of urgent treatment, a somewhat higher response rate (74%) was observed (which was the same as that for prednimustine) [23].

The rate of response is variable, but, in general, patients should not be evaluated until they have received interferon for at least 3 months. There are no published data with sufficiently long follow-up (given the natural history of follicular lymphoma) to know whether any of the remissions achieved with interferon as a single agent are in fact durable. With regard to toxicity, the majority of patients complain of flu-like symptoms with the first few injections but in almost everyone, the severity of these side-effects decreases with time. However, in patients receiving interferon for longer periods, e.g., one year, the majority feel noticably better on stopping the drug. In some patients, pre-medication with paracetamol can abrogate the initial side-effects.

Interferon in Combination with Other Drugs

By analogy with the principles of conventional cancer chemotherapy, having been investigated as a single agent, interferon was then combined with alkylating agents which are the mainstay of such conventional treatment for follicular lymphoma. The rationale for the combination was based on the results of experiments in murine L1210 leukaemia [24] and AKR lymphoma [25], which suggested synergy. Later studies in nude mice bearing human breast cancer xenografts once more demonstrated synergy between interferon and the drugs adriamycin and cyclophosphamide [26]. In the light of these results, albeit in a different disease, a study was carried out at St. Bartholomew's Hospital, London, combining chlorambucil given at conventional dose, with interferon given at low dose, thrice weekly, subcutaneously, in patients with low-grade lymphoma in whom conventional treatment had failed [27]. The combination was found to be feasible in terms of both clinical and haematological toxicity and responses were seen in 8/11 patients with follicular lymphoma, all of whom had received multiple previous therapies. Similar results have since been reported from other centres, patients receiving either chlorambucil or cyclophosphamide with 'low-dose interferon' (Table 2).

Table 2. Response rates with chemotherapy-interferon combinations

Treatment	CR+PR	No. pts.	Ref.
CB + IFN	8	11	[27]
CB + IFN	8	10	[28]
Cyclo + IFN	15	30	[29]
CB + IFN	27	49	[31]
CB + IFN	22	34	[30]

CB = chlorambucil; Cyclo = cyclophosphamide
IFN = interferon

Interferon has also been combined with drugs other than alkylating agents: in a second French study patients considered to have an urgent indication for treatment, i.e., those with large volume disease, were randomised to receive an adriamycin containing regimen, with or without interferon. In a preliminary analysis, the response rate was higher with the combination, although the follow-up is too short to know whether this will be reflected in prolongation of remission duration, or indeed survival [32].

In addition to studies in which interferon has been combined with standard drugs, a novel approach, based on the demonstration of synergy between interferon and anti-idiotype antibody therapy in a murine model, has been investigated at Stanford University. In 1986, Basham et al. reported responses in 8/16 patients with low-grade lymphoma who had been treated with anti-idiotype antibody alone [33]. Subsequently, Brown et al. (1989) reported a response rate of 9/12 in patients receiving both treatment modalities concurrently [34]. The studies are interesting but expensive and difficult to carry out in terms of defining the antibody to be used for each patient. Further results are awaited.

The activity of interferon as a single agent having been established and the combination with alkylating agent therapy having proven to be feasible, the next step was to compare the combination with conventional therapy. The encouraging results from St. Bartholomew's Hospital provided the rationale for a randomised comparison which is currently in progress in the United Kingdom: newly diagnosed patients with stage III or IV follicular lymphoma, in whom there is an indication for starting treatment, are randomised to receive either chlorambucil: 10 mg daily for 6 weeks, followed by 3, 2-week cycles, given at 14-day intervals, or chlorambucil as above, together with interferon 2 x 10^6 units/m^2 subcutaneously, thrice weekly throughout the 18-week period. Responding patients are then randomised again to receive no further therapy or 'maintenance' interferon for up to one year. The study thus attempts to answer 2 separate questions: first, does the addition of interferon to chlorambucil as initial therapy improve the response rate, and second, does the use of interferon as 'maintenance' therapy prolong remission duration? A similar study is being conducted in Italy [30]. The preliminary results of both can be summarised as follows: the addition of interferon to chlorambucil has not improved the response rate or the complete response rate. As expected, the combination is associated with a greater degree of myelosuppression than chlorambucil alone. However, significantly fewer relapses have been observed in patients receiving maintenance interferon, although as yet there is no survival advantage. In the British study, the 'best results' have been seen in the patients receiving interferon throughout [31].

Further support for the concept of interferon as maintenance comes from 2 other studies: at MD Anderson Hospital, patients have received more intensive initial therapy (comprising CHOP + bleomycin) followed by, in responding patients, interferon given as maintenance. Duration of remission was longer in comparison with that of a historical control group who had received the same initial therapy [35]. In an open study in Germany, patients in whom remission of follicular lymphoma had been achieved with conventional chemotherapy and who subsequently relapsed, received further chemotherapy to achieve a second complete or partial remission, which was then 'maintained' with interferon. In the majority, the duration of second remission was longer than that of the first [36]. The 4 studies described above have all used interferon as maintenance or continuation therapy. The concept is based to some degree on the original experiments in L1210 leukaemia which showed that the best results were obtained in mice in whom the amount of inoculated tumour was lowest [37]. Hence the hope that interferon might be useful in an adjuvant setting. Extrapolation has also been made from Strander's results in osteogenic sarcoma where interferon was given to children as adjuvant therapy following surgery in an attempt to prevent metastases [1].

The results are certainly encouraging but in the context of the natural history of follicular lymphoma, they are still preliminary and longer follow-up is required. Also, it is salutory to remember that the use of maintenance chemotherapy has, in the past, been shown to prolong remission duration in patients with follicular lymphoma, unfortunately without influencing survival [38].

Thus at present the data suggest that interferon may prolong remission, or perhaps more correctly, postpone recurrence. The difference is not purely a semantic one but based on the relatively low probability that interferons will actually cure patients with follicular lymphoma. This pessimistic view is based on the known difficulty of eradicating anything other than localised disease (which in some patients is curable with radiotherapy) [22,39-40], despite many attempts to do so with more [41,42] or less intensive chemotherapy [19-22], the use of total nodal or low-dose total body irradiation[43-45], and indeed, as mentioned above, maintenance chemotherapy [38]. However, it would be quite wrong to dismiss what has been achieved. A new treatment with perhaps a different mode of action from that of conventional cytotoxic chemotherapy certainly warrants further evaluation in carefully controlled clinical trials which are currently underway. It should be considered in the context of other new approaches that are being evaluated in follicular lymphoma, such as the drug fludarabine [46-48], and the use of myeloablative therapy with autologous bone marrow transplantation [49-52].

Cutaneous T-Cell Lymphoma

This is a rare disease characterised by clonal proliferation of mature helper (CD4+) T cells [53,54]. Patients usually present with red, plaque-like skin lesions which are relatively slow to progress but eventually the disease disseminates to involve lymph nodes and sometimes other organs. Conventional therapy (psoralen plus ultraviolet light [PUVA], topical nitrogen mustard and electron beam therapy) [55-57] is effective in the short term but responses are only very rarely more than temporary. Therefore, once more, a new approach is needed.

Systemic interferon alpha has been shown to be effective, often in patients who were refractory to all other forms of treatment, with response rates varying from 30-85% [58-64] and more recently, interferon-gamma has also been found to be useful [65] (Table 3). However, sustained complete remissions are rare. IFN-alpha has been investigated at both high and low doses in patients with both early and late stage disease. The total number of patients evaluable is still relatively small, thus the optimal dose remains unknown. There is, however, a suggestion of a dose/response relationship, the difficultly being that the majority of patients are unable to tolerate high doses for the length of time required to achieve the maximal response.

Table 3. Response rates with systemic interferon alpha and gamma treatment

	CR+PR	No. pts.	Ref.
IFN-α			
	9	20	[58]
	12	15	[59]
	15	22	[60]
	0	5	[61]
	17	20	[62]
	6	21	
	3	4	[64]
TOTAL	56 (65%)	86	
IFN-γ			
	5 (31%)	16	[65]

In Conclusion

There are a number of questions about the use of interferon which remain unanswered. Firstly, the mechanism of action has never been adequately elucidated. Gresser's experiments in L1210 leukaemia (using mouse interferon) clearly demonstrated what was considered to be a direct anti-proliferative effect [66]. The later experiments reported by Balkwill et al. (using human interferon) in nude mice bearing human cancer xenografts confirmed this, in view of the known species-specificity of interferon [26]. However, the situation is complicated by some seemingly conflicting data, also from Gresser et al., describing an experiment in which the growth of a transplantable L1210 leukaemia that was resistant to interferon *in vitro* was nonetheless inhibited *in vivo*, although to a lesser degree than that of a line that was known to be interferon sensitive [67]. The response was therefore interpreted as having been mediated by an immunological mechanism, invoking various possible cell types such as natural killer cells, the activity of which is enhanced by the presence of interferon. The controversy has never been settled.

The question of dose has also not been resolved. It is known that clinical toxicity becomes unacceptable for the majority of patients above a daily dose of 3-5 x 10^6 units and that high doses are not associated with greater responsiveness [17]. However, whether the most frequently used dose, i.e., 2 x 10^6 units thrice weekly, is actually necessary is unknown, it is possible that doses lower than this might be equally effective.

Finally, the drug has to be administered by injection with, on the whole, tolerable but sometimes appreciable side-effects.

As mentioned above, the majority of patients are relieved to have completed one year's maintenance therapy.

Thus the potential role of interferons remains to be determined fully. Certainly, they can induce regression of disease with a frequency similar to that of other treatment modalities. With currently available data it is difficult to justify the use of interferon as a single agent as the treatment of choice in newly diagnosed patients presenting with follicular or cutaneous T-cell lymphoma. Several studies are currently in progress which will hopefully answer the questions that remain.

Acknowledgement

I thank Claire Hole for typing the manuscript and Professor Andrew Lister for reading and improving it.

REFERENCES

1 Strander H, Cantell K, Carlstrom G et al: Clinical and laboratory investigations in man: systemic administration of potent IFN to man. JNCI 1973 (5):733

2 Quesada JR, Reuben J, Manning JT et al: Alpha interferon for induction of remission in hairy cell leukaemia. N Engl J Med 1984 (310):15-18

3 Golomb H, Fefer D, Golde D et al: Sequential evaluation of alpha-2b interferon treatment in 128 patients with hairy cell leukaemia. Semin Oncol 1988 (14):13

4 Ratain MJ, Golomb H, Vardiman J et al: Interferon alfa-2b therapy for hairy cell leukaemia in 69 patients. Blood 1989 (74):76(a)

5 Berman E, Heller G, Kempin S et al: Incidence of remission and long-term follow up in patients with hairy cell leukaemia treated with recombinant interferon alfa-2a. Blood 1990 (75):839-845

6 Talpaz M, Kantarijian HM, McCredie KB et al: Chronic myelogenous leukaemia: hematologic remission and cytogenetic improvements induced by recombinant alpha A interferon. N Engl J Med 1986 (314):1065-1069

7 Talpaz M, Kantarjian HM, McCredie KB et al: Clinical investigation of human alpha interferon in chronic myelogenous leukaemia. Blood 1987 (69):1280-1288

8 Giles FJ, Gray AG, Brozowic M et al: Alpha-interferon therapy for essential thrombocythaemia. Lancet 1988 (ii):70-72

9 Mandelli F, Avvisati G, Amadori S et al: Maintenance treatment with recombinant interferon alfa-2b in patients with multiple myeloma responding to conventional induction chemotherapy. N Engl J Med 1990 (322/20):1430-1434

10 Louie AC, Gallagher JC, Sikora K et al: Follow up observations on the effect of human leukocyte interferon in non-Hodgkin's lymphoma. Blood 1981 (58):712-718

11 Horning SJ, Merigan TC, Krown SE: Human interferon alpha in malignant lymphoma and Hodgkin's disease. Cancer 1985 (56):1305-1310

12 Gutterman JU, Blumenschein GR, Alexanian R: Leukocyte interferon-induced tumour regression in human metastatic breast cancer, multiple myeloma and malignant lymphoma. Ann Intern Med 1980 (93):399-406

13 Quesada GR, Hawkins M, Horning SJ et al: Collaborative phase I-II study of recombinant DNA-produced leukocyte interferon (clone A) in metastatic breast cancer, malignant lymphoma and multiple myeloma. Am J Med 1984 (77):427-432

14 O'Connell MJ, Colgan JP, Oken MM et al: Clinical trial of recombinant leukocyte A interferon as initial therapy for favourable histology non-Hodgkin's lymphomas and chronic lymphocytic leukaemia. J Clin Oncol 1986 (4): 128-136

15 Foon KA, Roth MS, Bunn PA: Interferon Therapy of non-Hodgkin's lymphoma. Cancer 1987 (59):601-604

16 Wagstaff J, Loynds P, Crowther D: A phase II study of human recombinant DNA-a2 interferon in patients with low-grade non-Hodgkin's lymphoma. Cancer Chemother Pharmacol 1986 (18):54-58

17 Foon KA, Sherwin SA, Abrams PG: Treatment of advanced non-Hodgkin's lymphoma with recombinant leukocyte A interferon.. N Engl J Med 1984 (311):1148-1152

18 Merigan TC, Sikora K, Bredden JE et al: Preliminary observations on the effect of human leukocyte interferon in non-Hodgkin's lymphoma. N Engl J Med 1978 (299):1449-1453.

19 Portlock CS et al: Treatment of advanced non-Hodgkin's lymphoma with favourable histology: preliminary results of a prospective trial. Blood 1976 (47):747

20 Lister TA, Cullen MH, Beard MET et al: Comparison of combined and single agent chemotherapy in non-Hodgkin's lymphoma of favourable histological subtype. Br J Med 1978 (1):533-537

21 Hoppe RT et al: The treatment of advanced stage favourable histology non-Hodgkin's lymphoma: A preliminary report of a randomised trial comparing single agent chemotherapy, combination chemotherapy and whole body irradiation. Blood 1981 (58):592-598

22 Gallagher CJ, Lister TA: Follicular non-Hodgkin's lymphoma. Baillieres Clin Haematol 1987 1(1):141-155

23 Solal-Seligny Ph, Lepage E, Brousse N et al: IFN-alpha 2b in patients with low tumour burden follicular non-Hodgkin's lymphoma. Preliminary results from the Groupe d'Etude des Lymphomes Folliculaires (GELF, France and Belgium). Suppl Eur J Cancer 1991 (in press)

24 Chirigos MA and Pearson JW: Cure of murine leukaemia with drugs and interferon treatment. JNCI 1973 (57):1367-1368

25 Gresser I, Maury C, Tovey M (1978). Efficacy of combined interferon cyclophosphamide therapy after diagnosis of lymphoma in AKR mice. Eur J Cancer 1978 (14):97-99

26 Balkwill FR and Moodie EM: Positive interactions between human interferon and cyclophosphamide or adriamycin in a human tumour model system. Cancer Res 1984 (44):904-908

27 Rohatiner AZS, Richards MA, Barnett MJ et al: Chlorambucil and interferon for low grade non-Hodgkin's lymphoma. Br J Cancer 1987 (55):225-226

28 Chisesi T, Capnist G, Vespignani M, Cetto G: Interferon alfa-2b and chlorambucil in the treatment

of non-Hodgkin's lymphoma. J Invest New Drugs 1987 (5):35
29 Ozer H, Anderson JR, Peterson BA et al: Combination trial of subcutaenous interferon alfa-2b and oral cyclophosphamide in favourable histology, non-Hodgkin's lymphoma. J Invest New Drugs 1987 (5):27
30 Chisesi T: Combination of interferon/chlorambucil therapy in low-grade non-Hodgkin's lymphoma. Suppl Eur J Cancer 1991 (in press)
31 Price CGA, Rohatiner AZS, Steward W et al: Interferon-alpha2b in the treatment of follicular lymphoma: preliminary results of a trial in progress. Ann Oncol 1991 (2 suppl 2):141-145
32 Celigny PS, Lepage E, Brousse N et al (1991). Interferon alfa-2b in patients with high tumour burden follicular non-Hodgkin's lymphoma. Preliminary results from the "Groupe D'Etude des Lymphomes Folliculaires" (GELF, France and Belgium). Suppl Eur J Cancer 1991 (in press)
33 Basham TY, Kaminski MS, Kitamura K, Levy R, Merigan TC: Synergistic antitumour effect of interferon and anti-idiotype monoclonal antibody in murine lymphoma. J Immunol 1986 (137/9):3019-3024
34 Brown SL, Miller RA, Horning S et al: Treatment of B cell lymphomas with anti-idiotype antibody therapy in combination with alpha interferon. Blood 1989 (73):651-661
35 McLaughlin P, Cabanillas F, Hagemeistr F et al: Alpha-interferon (IFN) prolongs remission in stage IV low grade lymphoma. Proc ASCO 1990 (9/267): abst 1034
36 Hiddemann W: Alpha interferon maintenance therapy in patients with low grade non-Hodgkin's lymphoma. Suppl Eur J Cancer 1991 (in press)
37 Gresser I, Bourali C, Levy JP et al: Increased survival in mice innoculated with tumour cells and treated with an IFN preparation. Proc Nat Acad Sci 1969 (63):51
38 Steward WP, Crowther D, McWilliam LJ et al: Maintenance chlorambucil after CVP in the management of advanced stage, low grade histologic type non-Hodgkin's lymphoma. Cancer 1988 (61/3):441-447
39 Paryani SB, Hoppe RT, Cox RS et al: Analysis of non-Hodgkin's lymphomas with nodular and favourable histologies, stages I and II. Cancer 1983 (52):2300
40 Richards MA, Gregory WM, Hall PA et al: Management of localised non-Hodgkin's lymphoma: the experience at St Bartholomew's Hospital 1972-1985. Haematol Oncol 1989 (7):1-18
41 McKelvey EM, Gottilev JA, Wilson HE et al: Hydroxydaunomycin (Adriamycin) combination chemotherapy in malignant lymphoma. Cancer 1975 (36/2): 428
42 Dana B, Dahlberge S, Miller T et al: Long term follow up of patients with low grade lymphoma treated with CHOP (cyclophosphamide, doxorubicin, vincristine, prednisolone) based chemotherapy or chemoimmunotherapy on Southwest oncology group studies. Proc ASCO 1989: abst 1001
43 Johnson RE, Canellos GP, Young RC et al: Chemotherapy (cyclophosphamide, vincristine and prednisolone) versus radiotherapy (total body irradiation) for stage III-IV poorly differentiated lymphocytic lymphoma. Cancer Treat Rep 1978 (62):321
44 Choi NC, Timothy AR, Kaufman SD: Low dose fractionated whole body irradiation in the treatment of advanced non-Hodgkin's lymphoma. Cancer 1979 (43): 1636
45 Hoppe RT, Kushlan P, Kaplan HS et al: The treatment of advanced stage favourable histology non-Hodgkin's lymphoma: a preliminary report of a randomised trial comparing single agent chemotherapy, combination chemotherapy and whole body irradiation. Blood 1981 (58):592
46 Leiby JM, Snider KM, Kraut EH et al: Phase II trial of 9-b-D-arabinosyl-2-fluoroadenine 5'-monophosphate in non-Hodgkin's lymphoma: prospective comparison of response with deoxycytidine kinase activity. Cancer Res 1987 (47):2719
47 Redman J, Cabanillas F, McLaughlin P et al: Fludarabine phosphate: a new agent with major activity in low grade lymphoma. Proc AACR 1988 (29):211
48 Hochster H and Cassileth P: Fludarabine phosphate therapy of non-Hodgkin's lymphoma. Semin Oncol 1990 (17):63-65
49 Schouten HC, Bierman PJ, Vaughan WP et al: Autologous bone marrow transplantation in follicular non-Hodgkin's lymphoma before and after histologic transformation. Blood 1989 (74):2579-2584
50 Colombat P, Desbois I, Biron P et al: Results of high dose chemotherapy with autologous bone marrow transplantation in 16 cases of follicular lymphoma. Exp Haematol 1989 (17):585
51 Freedman AS, Ritz J, Neuberg D et al: Autologous bone marrow transplantation in 69 patients with a history of low-grade B cell non-Hodgkin's lymphoma. Blood 1991 (in press)
52 Rohatiner AZS, Price CGA, Arnott S et al: Myeloablative therapy with autologous bone marrow transplantation as consolidation of remission in patients with follicular lymphoma. Ann Oncol 1991 (2):147-150
53 Epstein EH, Levin DL Croft JR et al: Mycosis fungoidis: survival, prognostic features, response to therapy and autopsy findings. Medicine 1972 (51):61-72
54 Haynes BF, Metzgar RS, Minna JD et al: Phenotypic characterisaton of cutaneous T cell lymphoma: Use of monoclonal antibodies to compare with other malignant T cell. N Engl J Med 1981 (304):1319-1323
55 Hamminga L, Hermans J, Noordijk EM et al: Cutaneous T cell lymphoma: Clinicopathological relationships, therapy and survial in 92 patients. Br J Dermatol 1982 (107):145-156
56 Vonderheid EC, Van Scott EJ, Wallner PE et al: A 10-year experience with topical mechlorethamine for mycosis fungoides: comparison with patients treated by total-skin electron-beam radiation therapy. Cancer Treat Rep 1979 (63):681-689
57 Winkler CF, Sausville EA, Ihde DC et al: Combined modality treatment of cutaneous T cell lymphoma:

Results of a 6 year follow up. J Clin Oncol 1986 (4):1094-1100
58 Bunn PA, Ihde DC, Foon KA: The role of recombinant interferon alpha-2a in the therapy of cutaneous T cell lymphomas. Cancer 1986 (57):1689-1695
59 Covelli A, Calvalieri R, Coppola G et al: Recombinant leukocyte A interferon (IFN-rA) as initial therapy in mycosis fungoides (MF) and Sezary syndrome (SS). Proc Am Soc Clin Oncol 1987 (6):189 (abst)
60 Olsen EA, Rosen ST, Vollmer RT et al: Interferon alpha-2a in the treatment of cutaneous T cell lymphoma. J Am Acad Dermatol 1989 (203):395-407
61 Thestrup-Pedersen K, Hammer R, Kaltoff K et al: Treatment of mycosis fungoides with recombinant interferon alpha-2a alone and in combination with etretinate. Br J Dermatol 1988 (118):811-818
62 Tura S, Mazza P, Zinzani PL et al: Alpha recombinant interferon in the treatment of mycosis fungoides. Hematologica 1987 (72):337-340
63 Ihde DC, Stays R, Sausville EA et al: A phase II trial of intermittent high dose recombinant interferon alpha-2a in mycosis fungoides and sezary syndrome. Proc AACR 1987:208
64 Vonderheid EC, Thompson R, Smiles KA et al: Recombinant interferon alfa-2b in plaque-phase mycosis fungoides. Intralesional and low dose intramuscular therapy. Arch Dermatol 1987 (123):757-763
65 Kaplan EH, Rosen ST, Norris DB et al: Phase II study of recombinant human interferon gamma for treatment of cutaneous T cell lymphoma. JNCI 1990 (82):208-212
66 Gresser I, Brouty-Boye D, Thomas M-T: Inhibition of the multiplication of mouse leukaemia L1210 cells in vitro by an IFN preparation. Proc Nat Acad Sci 1970 (66):1052
67 Gresser I, Maury C, Brouty-Boye D: Mechanism of the anti-tumour effect of IFN in mice. Nature 1972 (239):167

The Role of Interferons in Neuroendocrine Tumours and Aspects of Mechanisms of Action

Kjell E. Öberg

Ludwig Institute for Cancer Research and Department of Internal Medicine, University Hospital, 751 85 Uppsala, Sweden

Neuroendocrine tumours of the gastrointestinal tract and pancreas are rather rare tumours with an overall incidence of 0.9 per 100,000 people. The tumours derive from endocrine cells and are generally highly differentiated, showing production of various amines and peptides. Neuroendocrine tumours of the pancreas display clinical syndromes related to hormone production such as the Zollinger-Ellison syndrome due to increased gastrin secretion, hypoglycaemic symptoms due to insulin overproduction, and the glucagonoma syndrome due to glucagon production. There also exists a group of tumours, the so-called "non-functioning" tumours, which produce hormones that do not cause any definite clinical syndrome [1].

The most common type of neuroendocrine tumours in the gastrointestinal tract are the carcinoids which can be divided into fore-gut, mid-gut and hind-gut tumours. Mid-gut carcinoids are the most common, amounting to about 50% of all carcinoid tumours; the primary tumours are located in the jejunum, ileum, caecum or proximal colon. Patients with mid-gut carcinoids and liver metastases very often (75-80%) display the so called carcinoid syndrome, including flush, diarrhoea, bronchoconstriction and right heart failure [2]. These symptoms are related to increased secretion of serotonin, tachykinins and bradykinin from the tumours. Hind-gut carcinoids developing in the colon and rectum run a more indolent course, not displaying hormone-related clinical symptoms but more classical malignant signs such as bleeding and intestinal obstruction. The fore-gut type, which makes up about 20% of all carcinoid tumours, might develop in the thymus, bronchial, gastric or duodenal mucosa and displays a wide variety of clinical symptoms of endocrine diseases such as acromegaly, Cushing's disease or the Zollinger-Ellison syndrome with recurrent gastroduodenal ulcers.

The term malignant carcinoid syndrome is used when patients display the carcinoid syndrome with flush, diarrhoea, bronchoconstriction and/or right heart failure and also present increased excretion of 5-hydroxyindolacetic acid (5-HIAA) in the urine as well as liver metastases [3].

The median time from the onset of the first carcinoid symptoms to death is estimated at 8.6 years, with a wide range of 6-29 years. However, when patients display the malignant carcinoid syndrome with liver metastases, the median survival is 38 months if flushing occurs first, down to 14 months when high urinary excretion of 5-HIAA is recorded, and even less, i.e., 11 months, when the patient also has carcinoid heart disease [4,5].

Survival data concerning endocrine pancreatic tumours are relatively scarce. In 1950, Howard and colleagues reported on a large series of malignant insulinomas showing a median survival of 9.9 months from the onset of symptoms. With the advent of specific chemotherapy in the 1970s, mainly streptozotocin plus fluorouracil, the median survival increased more than 3-fold up to 36 months from the onset of symptoms (reviewed in [6]).

Previous Treatment

It is widely accepted that surgery should be considered as first-line treatment in most patients and even if total removal of the tumour is not possible debulking procedures might benefit the patient. Hepatic artery embolisation or ligation have been used with success in reducing hepatic metastases but these procedures do not cure the patient due to the possible development of collateral circulation within a couple of months (reviewed in [7]). Neuroendocrine tumours generally are not sensitive to irradiation but this therapy is mainly used to relieve pain from bone metastases. Medical treatment has 2 major aims: 1) to improve the symptoms by reducing hormone levels or block their peripheral action, and 2) to abrogate tumour growth.

Chemotherapy has been attempted since the early 1960s both as single agents and in combinations. The best results have been obtained with a combination of streptozotocin and 5-FU or doxorubicin. In malignant endocrine pancreatic tumours, objective responses are seen in 40-70% of patients, lasting for 1.5-2 years (6,8,9). However, only 10-30% of patients with carcinoid tumours show objective responses with the same combination and the responses are of very short duration, with a median of less than 6 months [10-12].

Somatostatin has been shown to inhibit symptoms related to neuroendocrine gut and pancreatic tumours and the long-acting analogue Sandostatin has a beneficial effect on these tumours [13,14]. Kvols and colleagues reported a significant decrease in hormone levels and clinical symptoms in about 70% of patients with the malignant carcinoid syndrome [15]. Antiproliferative effects by somatostatin analogues have not been documented.

Interferons

Interferons are normally occuring glycoproteins which can be induced during different conditions, e.g., infections. Antitumour effects have been demonstrated in a number of haematologic malignancies as well as in solid tumours [16,17]. Most commonly used are alpha-IFNs, both naturally occurring and recombinant forms. The reason for us to start treatment with alpha-IFN in 1982 was the observation that patients with neuroendocrine tumours showed decreased natural killer cell activity. As alpha-IFN is a well-known stimulator of NK cell activity we started to use human leukocyte interferon in patients with malignant neuroendocrine gut and pancreatic tumours. Even if the primary observation was false, significant effects on circulating hormone levels and clinical symptoms were observed, which encouraged us to continue these trials [18]. Since then, multiple studies with alpha-IFNs in the treatment of malignant endocrine gut and pancreatic tumours were published [6,18-22]. The overall biochemical response rates were about 50%, with significant tumour reduction in 15-20% of patients. A limited number of patients with malignant neuroendocrine tumours were treated with a combination of alpha and gamma-IFN [23]. Local intratumoral application of beta-IFN in a small number of patients has also been performed [24].

Endocrine Pancreatic Tumours - Therapy with Alpha Interferon

A total of 32 patients with different endocrine pancreatic tumours: Zollinger-Ellizon syndrome (n=5), WDHA syndrome (n=10), "non-functioning" tumours (n=14), insulinoma (n=2) and glucagonoma (n=1), and liver metastases were treated subcutaneously with doses of 3-9 million units per day (median 6 MU/day) of human leukocyte interferon or recombinant interferon-alpha 2b. All patients were treated after failure on chemotherapy with streptozotocin plus 5-FU or doxorubicin. More than 50% reduction in biochemical markers was obtained in 20 out of 32 patients (63%), whereas a more than 50% decrease in tumour size was obtained in 7 patients (21%). Stabilisation of the disease was noted in 5 cases (16%) and tumour progression in 7 (21%). In relation to decreasing circulating hormone levels the clinical symptoms were reduced or even disappeared. Subjective response was obtained in 24 patients (75%). The median duration of objective response was 20.5 months (2-37 mo) [16]. Figure 1 illustrates the effect of alpha-IFN on circulating hormone levels in a patient with a glucagonoma and Figure 2a and b illustrate the effects on tumour size in a patient with gastrinoma. The treatment was equally effec-

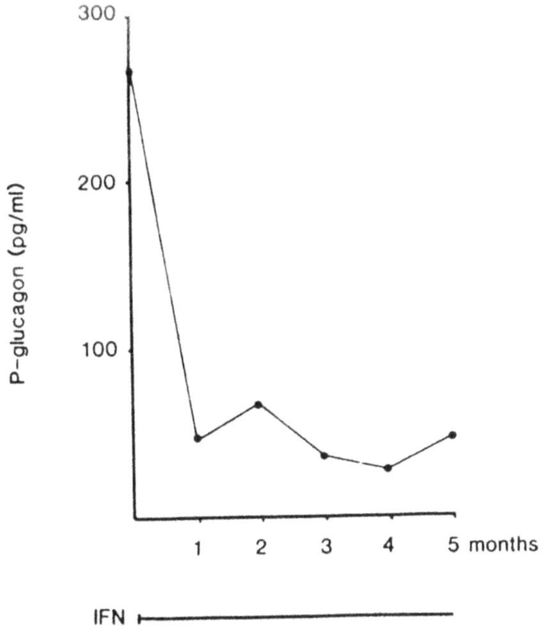

Fig. 1. Effects of alpha-IFN on plasma glucagon in a patient with a glucagon-producing endocrine pancreatic tumour

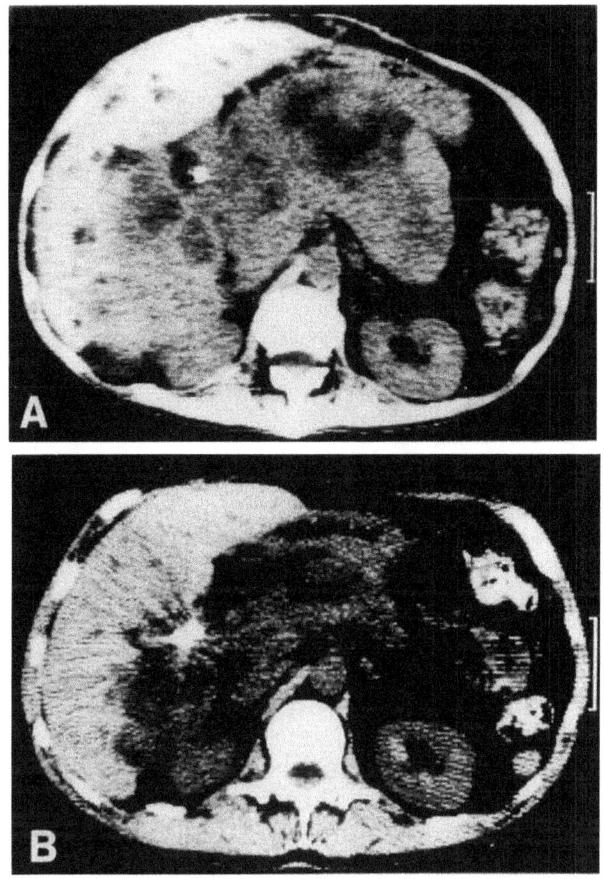

Fig. 2. Patient with a gastrin-producing endocrine pancreatic tumour previous to start of alpha-IFN therapy (Fig. 2A) and after 6 months of IFN treatment (Fig. 2B)

tive in functioning as well as "non-functioning" endocrine pancreatic tumours.
In conclusion, alpha-IFN seems to be at least as effective as chemotherapy (streptozotocin plus 5-FU) in the management of patients with malignant neuroendocrine pancreatic tumours.

Carcinoid Tumours - Therapy with Alpha Interferon

Carcinoid tumours are more frequent than endocrine pancreatic tumours and also present more uniform clinical symptoms, i.e., the carcinoid syndrome. Therefore, more clinical studies with alpha-IFN therapy have been performed in carcinoid tumour patients. Our first study, published in 1983 [18], clearly demonstrated that alpha-IFN had a significant impact on circulating hormone levels and clinical symptoms. Since then, a total of 130 patients with histologically varified malignant carcinoid tumours and liver metastases were referred to our unit for treatment. One group, consisting of 19 patients (Group A), was admitted before 1982 and therefore received streptozotocin plus 5-FU as the only treatment

Another group, of 68 patients (Group B), received chemotherapy as first-line treatment and after failure alpha-IFN. A third group, consisting of 43 patients (Group C), received alpha-IFN as first-line and only treatment. The majority of the patients, 75% in all groups, had the primary tumour located in the mid-gut region and the median age at diagnosis was 58 years. Median urinary 5-hydroxy-indolacetic acid (5-HIAA) at the start of treatment was 569, 559 and 390 μmol/24h, respectively, which indicated that there was no significant difference between the 3 groups of patients regarding clinical parameters. In total, 111 patients received alpha-IFN subcutaneously, 73 patients were treated with human leukocyte interferon at doses of 2-6 MU 7 times per week (median 6 MU 7 times/w), 38 patients were treated with recombinant interferon-alpha 2b (Intron A) at doses of 3-9 MU

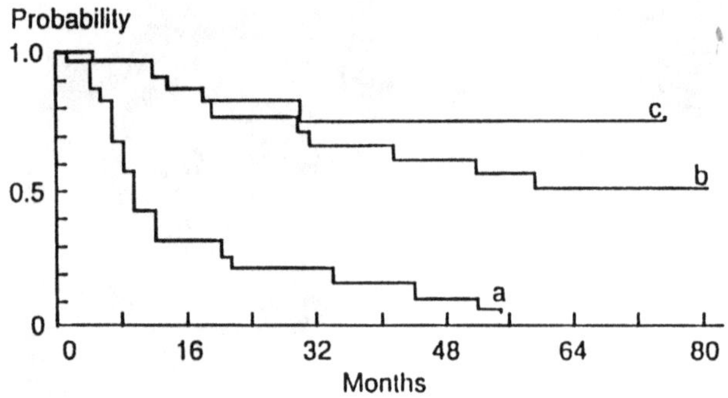

Fig. 3. Probability of survival from start of treatment in 3 different groups of patients with malignant carcinoid tumours. Group A (n=19) received only chemotherapy (streptozocin + 5-FU), in Group B (n=68) the patients started on chemotherapy and subsequently received alpha-IFN when tumour progression occurred, Group C (n=43) received alpha-IFN from the beginning. Kaplan-Meier analysis showed Group C vs A $p < 0.001$

3-5 times/w, median 5 MU 3 times/w. The median duration of interferon therapy was 30 months with a range of 3-66 months. Those patients receiving chemotherapy (Group A and Group B) were given streptozotocin 1 g for 5 days combined with 5-FU 400 mg/m^2 intravenously as induction, followed by a maintenance bolus dose of 2 g streptozotocin plus 400 mg/m^2 5-FU intravenously every 3 weeks.

Fourty-seven out of 111 patients (42%) treated with alpha-IFN (Groups B+C) showed an objective response in biochemical markers and among these 16 (14%) had a more than 50% reduction in tumour size. Disease stabilisation was seen in 43 patients (39%) while 21 (19%) showed progressive disease. The median duration of response was 34 months (range 3-66 months). Subjective responses with lessening of diarrhoea, flush and bronchoconstriction were noticed in 76 patients (68%). Two out of 19 patients treated with chemotherapy (Group A) showed an objective response (10%), both with biochemical responses which lasted for 3 and 5 months, respectively. Seven patients had stable disease for a median of 5 months while 10 patients progressed. Survival analysis (Kaplan-Meier) showed a median survival from the start of treatment of 8 months in the group of patients treated with chemotherapy alone (Group A), whereas the median survival in the group of patients treated with alpha-IFN alone (Group C) was 80+ months ($p < 0.001$). In Group B, i.e., patients who had received chemotherapy followed by alpha-IFN, the median survival was 64 months (Fig. 3). There was no significant difference in survival between Groups B and C. The 5- and 10-year survival rates from diagnosis in our interferon-treated patients were 80%.

In a study by Moertel and colleagues from the Mayo Clinic [25] who used higher doses of alpha-IFN 2a (Roferon), median 24 x 10 MU/m^2/day subcutaneously, similar objective response rates were obtained in 27 patients with metastatic carcinoid tumours. Thirty-nine percent of the patients showed biochemical responses and 20% a significant reduction in tumour size. The duration of treatment was short (median 28 days) because of considerable adverse reactions against alpha-IFN treatment. Subjective responses were seen in 65% of patients.

In a recent study by Hansen and colleagues [26], 46 patients with histologically confirmed mid-gut carcinoid tumours and liver metastases were treated daily with 5 MU alpha-IFN 2b (Intron A) subcutaneously for a period of up to 2 years. In a number of patients the treatment was combined with embolisation of the hepatic arteries and they found that when interferon was given alone, 24% of patients responded biochemically, 43% had stable disease while 19% progressed. The survival rate was 40% at 5 years from the start of treatment. The median survival time from the start of treatment was 3 years and 4 months. When embolisation of the liver arteries had been performed prior to the start of interferon treatment the biochemical response rate increased to 60%, 20% had stable disease and 20% progressed after 1 year. The survival rate was 75% after 5 years of observation. The authors conclude that interferon is an effective treatment for malignant metastatic mid-gut carcinoids and that embolisation prior to start of alpha-IFN improves both response rates and survival.

In a recent randomised controlled study recombinant IFN-alpha 2a alone was compared with recombinant IFN-alpha 2a plus streptozotocin plus doxorubicin [27]. A total of 22 patients with malignant carcinoid tumours were enrolled, 12 were randomised to alpha-IFN alone (Group A), 10 to alpha-IFN plus chemotherapy (Group B). The dose of alpha-

IFN was 3 MU/m^2 x 3/w and streptozotocin was given as a bolus injection of 2g and doxorubicin 40 mg/m^2 every 3 weeks. There was no statistical difference in the response rates between the 2 groups: Group A: 1 CR, 9 SD, 2 PD; Group B: 10 SD. However, considerable toxicity was noticed in the chemotherapy arm (Group B). One patient died from doxorubicin myocardial toxicity despite a doxorubicin dose of less than 50% of the suggested toxicity dose. After 6 months of therapy 20 patients were switched to single-drug therapy with IFN-alpha 2a 3 MU/m^2 x 5/w for another 6 months. The biochemical response rate increased to 5 PR, 14 SD and 1 PD. Tumour size remained unchanged throughout the observation period.

These response rates were somewhat lower than could be expected with alpha-IFN but might be explained by the high frequency of neutralising interferon antibodies (see below).

Twelve patients, 5 women and 7 men with malignant carcinoid tumours who had been treated with alpha-IFN for at least 6 months and showed stable or progressive disease, were selected for combination treatment with natural gamma-IFN (Finnish Red Cross). The dose of alpha-IFN was 5-10 MU s.c. 3-5 times/w plus gamma-IFN 0.5-1.0 MU s.c. daily. A biochemical response was noted in 1 patient while 7 showed stable disease and 4 progressed. No reduction in tumour size was noticed. The side-effects were similar to those of alpha-IFN alone but additive. We conclude that this regimen showed little or no benefit to this group of patients with advanced stages of disease. However, an antitumoral effect cannot be ruled out when alpha-IFN and gamma-IFN are combined from the start of treatment in patients with less advanced stages of disease [23].

Five patients, 3 with mid-gut carcinoids, 1 with lung carcinoid and 1 with endocrine pancreatic tumour, all with advanced stages of disease and large liver metastases, were included in a study with beta-IFN. The patients had previously been treated with alpha-IFN and somatostatin analogue. Natural beta-interferon (AP-Medical, Germany) was injected under ultrasound guidance once a week directly into one of the largest liver metastases in 4 patients and into 3 different metastases in one. The doses were 9-15 MU per injection disposed uniformly in the tumours. The patients received 4-12 courses. Two of the 3 patients with mid-gut carcinoids showed a biochemical response but the responses were short lasting (3-4 weeks). The patient with lung carcinoid progressed while the patient with endocrine pancreatic tumour remained stable. All patients experienced subjective improvement. The adverse reactions were similar to those of alpha-IFNs. Beta-interferon given locally seems to be effective in neuroendocrine tumours. However, the local treatment must be combined with systemic therapy to obtain more long-lasting responses [24].

Adverse Reactions

The adverse effects of alpha-IFN treatment are well-known to most readers [28]. They include flue-like symptoms (89%), fatigue (40%), weight loss (59%), and reduction of peripheral blood counts (30%). Most of these adverse events were mild (WHO 1-2) and could be managed by dose adjustments. Disturbed lipid metabolism with increased serum triglycerides were noticed in 32% of patients and development of liver steatosis in 11%. A number of patients (19%) developed autoimmune diseases, complications which are not so well described in the literature. Most patients presented thyroid dysfunctions with both hypo- and hyperthyroidism, one patient developed an SLE syndrome and 2 patients autoimmune vasculitis. Exacerbation of psoriasis was also noticed in some patients [29,30].

Anti-interferon antibodies developed in a number of patients receiving recombinant alpha-IFNs. Patients treated with human leukocyte interferon (n=81) did not display any neutralising interferon antibodies but one patient had low titre of binding antibodies. However, in patients treated with recombinant interferon-alpha 2b, Intron A (n=151), 4% neutralising interferon antibodies and 12% binding antibodies were observed. Even higher frequencies were noticed in patients treated with recombinant interferon 2a (Roferon) (n=26) with neutralising interferon antibodies in 27% and binding in 31% of the

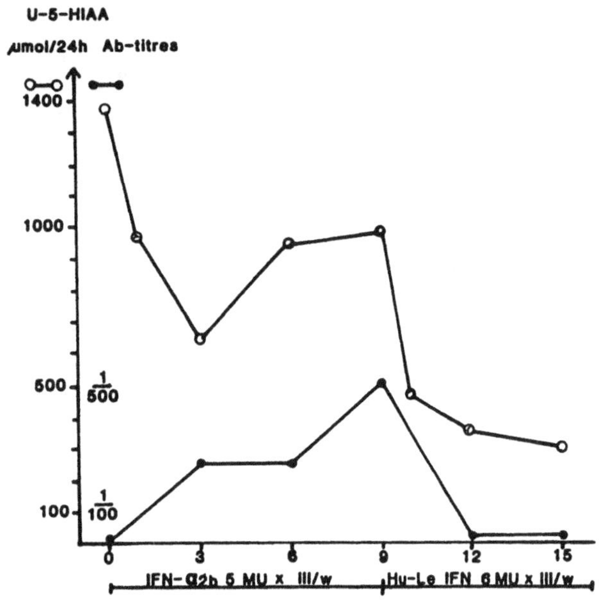

Fig. 4. Patient treated with recombinant alpha-IFN 2b developing neutralising interferon antibodies. Note the disappearance of biochemical response in parallel with ab-formation and regain of response after change to human leukocyte IFN

patients. More than half of the patients who developed neutralising interferon antibodies presented concomittant loss of biochemical response and a change to human leukocyte interferon could restore the clinical antitumour response [20] (Fig. 4).

Mechanisms of Action of Alpha Interferons

Treatment with alpha-IFNs in patients with neuroendocrine tumours has revealed some important findings. Firstly, most objective responses were obtained in biochemical markers whereas a considerably less significant reduction of tumour size has been observed. The study by Hanson et al. [26] also suggested that tumour mass might have an impact on the therapeutic results. Reduction in tumour size by pretreatment with embolisation of liver metastases significantly improved the objective response rates. Secondly, a large group of patients showed stabilisation of the disease without any further growth of the tumour and abrogation of hormone secretion. Such stabilisation might have influenced the quality of life and long-term survival. Traditional response criteria such as complete and partial remissions related to decrease in tumour size have not been quite appropriate in evaluating patients on biotherapy. Even when only partial remisions were obtained, mostly biochemically and not related to tumour size, significant improvement in quality of life as well as high survival rates have been noted compared to historical material of patients treated with chemotherapy. The median survival from the start of treatment was 8-12 months for patients with malignant carcinoid tumours treated with chemotherapy compared to 60-80 months in material of patients on alpha-IFN therapy. These data need to be confirmed in forthcoming randomised controlled studies.

A third important observation is the development of autoimmunity in about 25% of the patients. One patient who developed an SLE syndrome obtained a complete remission 2 years after withdrawal of alpha-IFN treatment. Explorative laparotomy 1 year later showed no signs of remaining tumour tissue. In this particular patient development of an autoimmune reaction might have caused the complete remission. However, in extensive patient material (n=135) no correlation was found between antitumour responses and development of autoimmune diseases [29]. Possible development of neutralising interferon antibodies has to be followed because of the risk of concomitant loss of antitumour effects. Changes from recombinant alpha-INFs to human leukocyte interferon might be of benefit to such patients. The observed differences in the ability to develop neutralising interferon antibodies between the different recombinant alpha-IFN preparations need further clarification.

The mechanism of action of alpha-IFNs in various tumours has yet to be elucidated. We can demonstrate in neuroendocrine tumours that the cell cycle is blocked in the G0, G1 phase [31], and that specimens from tumours of patients treated with alpha-IFN show significantly lower proliferative activity measured with the antibody Ki-67, a proliferation marker. In parallel with this increased proliferation rate, decreased expression of mRNA

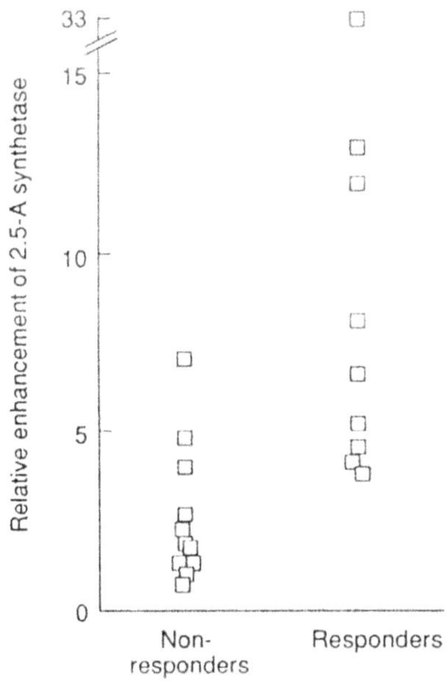

Fig. 5. Induction of 2-5 A-synthetase in tumour cells *in vitro* from patients with malignant carcinoid tumours. There was a significant correlation between *in vitro* induction of 2-5 A synthetase and clinical response ($p < 0.01$)

for various hormones and growth factors has been demonstrated [32]. Such decrease in mRNA expression might have been regulated on a post-transcriptional level and possibly by induction of 2'-5' A-synthetase and P68 kinases. We have been able to demonstrate a relation between biochemical responses and induction of 2'-5' A-synthetase in tumour cells from carcinoid tumour patients [33] (Fig. 5). Furthermore, biopsy specimens taken regularly from patients during alpha-IFN treatment showed increasing amounts of fibrous tissue and decreasing numbers of tumour cells with time [34] (Fig. 6). Thus, alpha-IFN seemed to induce tumour fibrosis, a phenomenon which has also been noticed in nude mice models with human tumour xenographs from osteosarcoma treated with alpha-IFN [34]. Such increased fibrosis seemed not to be induced by increased expression of known growth factors like PDGF or EGF [36]. These growth factors are expressed in the stroma and in carcinoid tumour cells but the expression is not enhanced by alpha-IFN treatment.

Most data indicate that alpha-IFN exerts direct effects on neuroendocrine tumour cells and that these might be the most important mechanisms of action. However, increased expression of class I antigen has been obtained in tumour specimens after alpha-IFN treatment in patients with carcinoid tumours, indicating that the immune system might play a role [37].

It has become evident from our studies that alpha-IFN treatment must be continued for very long periods of time and that patients are

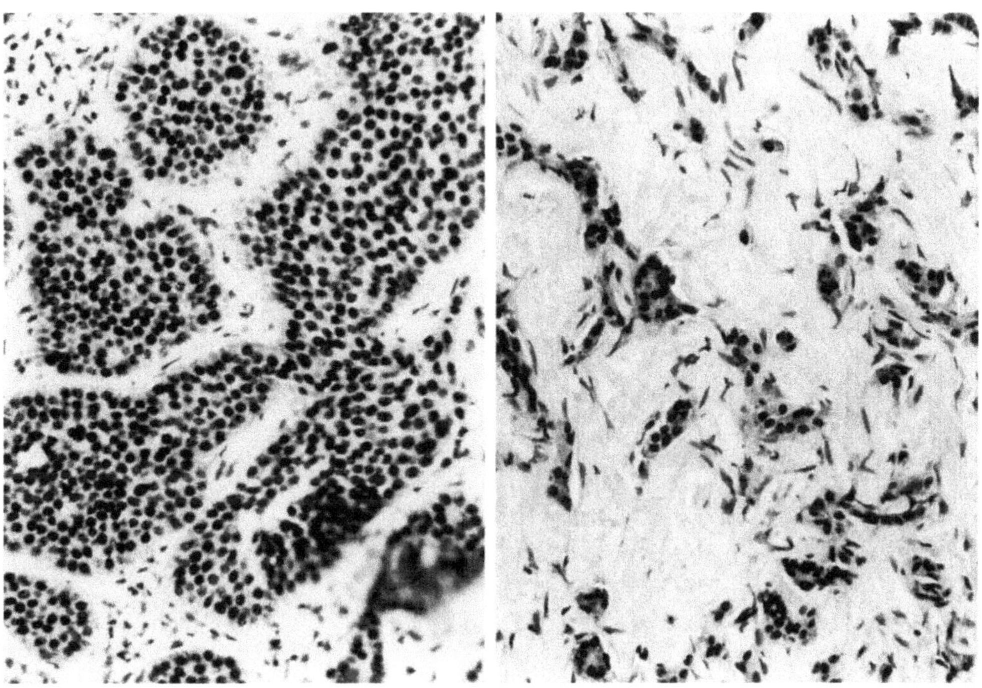

Fig. 6. Induction of fibrosis in liver metastases from a patient with carcinoid tumour. The left panel shows the tumour growth pattern previous to alpha-IFN treatment and the right panel after 6 months of therapy. Note the reduction in tumour cells and increased fibrosis

not cured by this type of treatment. When the therapy was withdrawn for whatever reason, progression of the disease occurred within 6-12 months. An important observation has been that the patient is not resistant to alpha-IFN after such withdrawal and the treatment can be re-introduced with similar objective therapy responses. There are also indications that low to moderate doses of alpha-IFN should be used to increase the tolerability and make treatment possible for long periods of time.

Conclusion

Alpha interferons have clearly demonstrated antitumour activity in neuroendocrine tumours, with significant effects on biochemical markers, clinical symptoms and possibly also impact on survival. However, the latter has to be proved in randomised controlled studies. Alpha interferons seemed to have direct antitumour effects but involvement of the immune system could not be ruled out. *In vitro* testing of induction of 2'-5' A-synthetase in tumour cells might predict clinical outcome and sort out patients resistant to alpha-IFN treatment. Low to moderate doses of alpha-IFN should be used for long periods of time and the patient should be monitored for development of autoimmune reactions as well as neutralising interferon antibodies, the latter when recombinant interferons are used. Typical clinical signs of development of neutralising interferon antibodies were disappearance of side-effects such as fatigue and malaise and increasing leukocyte counts. So far, the combination of alpha-IFN with chemotherapy has not demonstrated any beneficial effect compared to alpha-IFN alone. On the contrary, more severe adverse reactions were observed. However, combination with other biotherapies, somatostatin analogues, gamma-IFN and beta-IFN need to be further analysed.

REFERENCES

1 Eriksson B, Öberg K, Andersson T, Arnberg H, Lindgren PG, Lörelius LE, Lundqvist G, Magnusson A, Wide L, Wilander E: Neuroendocrine pancreatic tumours: clinical presentation, biochemical and histopathological findings in 84 patients. J Int Med 1990 (228):103-113

2 Norheim I, Öberg K, Theodorsson-Norheim E et al: Malignant carcinoid tumours; An analysis of 103 patients with regard to tumour localization, hormone production and survival. Ann Surg 1987 (206):115-125

3 Davis Z, Moertel CG, Mc Ilrath DC: The malignant carcinoid syndrome. Surg Gynecol Obstet 1973 (137):637-644

4 Goodwin JD: Carcinoid tumors: An analysis of 2837 cases. Cancer 1975 (36): 560-569

5 Moertel CG, Sauer WG, Dockerty MB, Baggentoss AH: Life history of the carcinoid tumor of the small intestine. Cancer 1961 (14): 901-912

6 Eriksson B, Skogseid B, Lundqvist G, Wide L, Wilander E, Öberg K: Medical treatment and long-term survival in a prospective study of 84 patients with endocrine pancreatic tumors. Cancer 1990 (65): 1883-1890

7 Moertel CG: An odyssey in the land of small tumors. J Clin Oncol 1987 (5): 1503

8 Moertel CG, Hanley JA, Johnsson LA: Streptozocin alone compared with streptozocin plus fluorouracil in the treatment of advanced islet cell carcinoma. N Engl J Med 1980 (303): 1189-1194

9 Öberg K, Eriksson B: Medical treatment of neuroendocrine gut and pancreatic tumors. Acta Oncol 1989 (28): 425-431

10 Öberg K, Norheim I, Lundqvist G, Wide L: Cytotoxic treatment in patients with malignant carcinoid tumors. Respons to streptozocin alone or in combination with 5-FU. Acta Oncol 1987 (26): 429-432

11 Norheim I, Öberg K, Alm G: Treatment of malignant carcinoid tumors; a randomized controlled study of streptozocin plus 5-FU and human leucocyte interferon. Eur J Cancer Clin Oncol 1989 (25):1475-1479

12 Moertel CG, Hanley JA: Combination therapy trials in metastatic carcinoid tumors and the malignant carcinoid syndrome. Cancer Clin Trials 1970 (2): 327-334

13 Eriksson B, Öberg K, Andersson T et al: Treatment of malignant endocrine pancreatic tumours with a new long acting somatostatin analogue SMS 201-995. Scand J Gastroenterol 1988 (23):508

14 Öberg K, Norheim I, Lundqvist G, Wide L: Treatment of the carcinoid syndrome with SMS 201-995, a somatostatin analogue. Scand J Gastroenterol 1986 (21):191-192

15 Kvols LK, Moertel CG, O'Connell MS et al: Treatment of malignant carcinoid syndrome evaluation of a long acting somatostatin analogue. New Engl J Med 1986 (315): 663-666

16 Quesada JR, Talpaz M, Gutterman JU: Interferons in hematological malignancies. In: Baron S, Dianzani R, Stanton GJ, Fleischman WR Jr (eds) The Interferon System. University of Texas Press, Austin 1987 pp 486-495

17 Bonnem E: Interferon: Potential use in solid tumours. In: Baron S, Dianzani R, Stanton GJ, Fleischman WR Jr (eds) The Interferon System. University of Texas Press, Austin 1987 pp 506-516

18 Öberg K, Funa K, Alm G: Effects of leukocyte interferon on clinical symptoms and hormone levels in patients with mid-gut carcinoid tumors and carcinoid syndrome. N Engl J Med 1983 (309): 129-133

19 Öberg K, Norheim I, Lind E. et al: Treatment of malignant carcinoid tumors with human leukocyte interferon. Long-term results. Cancer Treatm Rep 1986 (70):1297-1304

20 Öberg K, Alm G, Magnusson A, Lundqvist G, Theodorsson E, Wide L, Wilander E: Treatment of malignant tumors with recombinant interferon alpha-2b (Intron-A); Development of neutralizing interferon and possible loss of antitumor activity. JNCI 1989 (81): 531-535

21 Eriksson B, Öberg K, Alm G, et al: Treatment of malignant endocrine pancreatic tumours with human leukocyte interferon. Lancet 1986 (2): 1307-1309

22 Öberg K, Lindström H, Alm G, Lundqvist G: Successful treatment of therapy-resistant pancreatic cholera with human leukocyte interferon. Lancet 1985 (1):725-727

23 Tiensuu Janson E, Kauppinen HL, Öberg K: A phase II trial with alpha-IFN and natural gamma-IFN in patients with advanced stages of malignant carcinoid tumours. J Interferon Res 1990 (10 suppl 1):128

24 Tiensuu Janson E, Andersson T, Öberg K: Local ß-interferon treatment in patients with neuroendocrine gut and pancreatic tumours - A preliminary report. J Interferon Res 1990 (10 suppl 1):128

25 Moertel C, Rubin J, Kvols LK: Therapy of metastatic carcinoid tumor and the malignant carcinoid syndrome with recombinant leucocyte A interferon. J Clin Oncol 1989 (7):865-868

26 Hansen L-E, Schrumpt E, Jacobsen MB, Kolbenstvedt AN, Kolmannskog F, Bergur A, Dolva LO: The extended experience with recombinant alpha-2b interferon with or without hepatic artery embolization in the treatment of mid-gut carcinoid tumors. Acta Oncol 1991 (in press)

27 Tiensuu Janson E, Alm G, Grandér D, Öberg K: A randomized controlled study of gamma-IFN alpha 2a vs gamma-IFN alpha 2a and chemotherapy in malignant carcinoid disease. J Interferon Res 1990 (10 suppl 1):127

28 Quesada JR, Talpaz M, Rios A, Kurzrock R, Gutterman JU: Clinical toxicity of interferons in cancer patients: a review. J Clin Oncol 1986 (4): 234-243

29 Rönnblom L, Alm G, Öberg K: Automimmunity in carcinoid patients treated with alpha-interferon. Ann Int Med 1991 (in press)

30 Burman P, Tötterman HT, Öberg K, Karlsson FA: Thyroid autoimmunity in patients on long-term therapy with leucocyte-derived interferon. J Clin Endocrinol Metabol 1986 (ii):1307-1309

31 Wilander E, Bengtsson A, Norheim I, Öberg K, Brodin E: Interferon-induced nuclear DNA

alterations in malignant carcinoid tumours in vivo. JNCI 1986 (76):429-433

32 Funa K, Eriksson B, Wilander E, Öberg K: Expression of chromogranin A and B mRNA in carcinoid tumors studied by in situ hybridization. Endocrinol (in press)

33 Grandér D, Öberg K, Lundqvist M-L et al: Interferon-induced enhancement of 2'-5'-oligoadenylate synthetase in mid-gut carcinoid tumors. Lancet 1990 (336): 337-340

34 Andersson T, Wilander E, Eriksson B, Lindgren PG, Öberg K: Effects of interferon on tumor tissue content in liver metastases of carcinoid tumors. Cancer Res 1990 (50): 3413-3415

35 Brosjö O, Bauer HCF, Broström LÅ, et al: Influence of human alpha-interferon on four human osteosarcoma xenografts in nude mice. Cancer Res 1985 (45): 5598-5602

36 Funa K, Papanicolaou V, Juhlin C, Rastad J, Åkerström G, Heldin EH, Öberg K: Expression of platelet-derived growth factor ß-receptors on stromal tissue cells in carcinoid tumours. Cancer Res 1990 (50): 748-753

37 Funa K, Gazdar AF, Doyle A et al: In vivo induction of ß2 microglobulin after interferon therapy on small-cell lung cancer and mid-gut carcinoid patients. Clin Immunol Immunopathol 1986 (41): 159-164

The Interferons plus Other Modalities of Cancer Therapy

John Wagstaff

Department of Medical Oncology, Free University Hospital, De Boelelaan 1117, 1007 MB Amsterdam, The Netherlands

The year 1990 marked the tenth anniversary of the introduction of the recombinant alpha-interferons (IFN-alpha) into clinical trial. Although not fulfilling the expectations of the media that they would be the panacea for cancer, they have become an essential adjunct to the management of a number of human malignancies. The current thrust of clinical development of the IFNs is moving away from single agent usage and towards combined modality programmes incorporating other cytokines, monoclonal antibodies and chemotherapeutic agents. Single agent maintenance therapy with interferon, once a low volume disease state has been achieved by other treatments, is another approach which is proving to be of some value. The aim of this chapter is, therefore, to discuss the available data relating to the use of the IFNs in combination with these other treatment modalities.

Interferons and Chemotherapy

During the past years the IFNs have undergone extensive testing in a wide variety of human malignancies. In relatively few is single agent IFN currently regarded as first-line therapy. Examples may include hairy cell leukaemia and some of the myeloproliferative diseases. In other diseases such as renal cell carcinoma, multiple myeloma and malignant melanoma, a small proportion of the patients will respond but usually only for a relatively short period of time. A large number of cancers, including some of the most common adult solid tumours, do not respond at all to the IFNs. On the other hand, chemotherapy can achieve remissions in a high proportion of patients with cancers such as breast cancer and small cell lung cancer, but these patients virtually always relapse, become resistant and die of their disease. The unique biological properties of the IFNs suggest that it may be of value to combine these agents with chemotherapy even though the IFN itself may not be active in that particular tumour type.

When an IFN is active in its own right it may add to or synergise with the antitumour effects of chemotherapy by operating through a different mechanism. Toxicity may not be exacerbated because the IFNs possess a different spectrum of toxicity to those of cytotoxic agents. The IFNs may also be usefully combined with chemotherapy, even when they are inactive as single agents, by modulating the interaction between the cytotoxic agent and either the tumour cells or the host. IFNs may alter the phenotype of the tumour cells, thus making them more susceptible, or they may perturb the patient's metabolism, thus altering the pharmacokinetics or pharmacodynamics of the chemotherapeutic agents.

These putative interactions have led to the conduct of a number of tissue culture and animal experiments, the results of which suggest that combinations of the IFNs and chemotherapy may have additive or synergistic antitumour activity. In tissue culture, positive interactions were seen between IFNs and drugs such as doxorubicin (Dox), cisplatinum (CDDP), actinomycin-D, etoposide and 5-fluorouracil (5-FU) [reviewed in 1,2].

Anthracyclines

One of the major mechanisms of drug resistance is related to the ability of resistant tumour cells to extrude drug from the cell by utilising the P glycoprotein pump. Cells which develop resistance through this mechanism are generally resistant to a number of structurally unrelated drugs which include the anthracyclines, the vinca alkaloids and etoposide. The interferons have been studied for their ability to reverse the MDR phenotype and have not been shown to be capable of doing this. However, a recent study [3] demonstrated that in 3 cell lines the intracellular concentration of Dox was increased when the cells were simultaneously exposed to IFN-beta or IFN-gamma. This was translated into an additive effect of the combination on cell growth. Similar growth inhibitory effects were seen on the same cell lines growing in nude mice and treated with 5000 IU IFN-gamma plus 5 or 25 µg of Dox twice per week. This phenomenon was not, however, mediated via interaction with the P glycoprotein pump since drug efflux was not affected by the IFN treatment.

Two phase I studies [4,5] have investigated Dox given every 3 weeks together with IFN-alpha given either at 10 mU/m^2 x3/week for 2 weeks or 12 mU/m^2/day x 5 days. The maximum tolerable dose (MTD) for Dox in both of these studies was 30 to 40 mg/m^2 and the dose limiting toxicity was myelosuppression. This Dox dose is approximately 50% less than it is possible to administer as a single agent, indicating that toxicity was at least additive. Two other groups [6,7] gave the IFN-alpha continuously 3 times per week at 10 mU/m^2 and the Dox weekly. In this scheduling the dose recommended for phase II evaluation was 25 mg/m^2/week which is equivalent to the Dox dose used as a single agent. In one of these 2 latter studies [6], hepatic toxicity was observed and because the anthracyclines are metabolised by the liver this suggested that an interaction may be occurring via perturbation of the metabolism of the anthracycline. Eksborg et al. [8] studied the pharmacokinetics of epirubicin 100 mg/m^2 either with or without IFN 6 mU/day and were unable to demonstrate any alteration.

These data taken together suggest that weekly Dox at a dose of 25 mg/m^2 together with 5-10 mU/m^2 IFN-alpha 3 times per week is the optimal schedule for further evaluation in phase II and III studies.

Alkylating Agents

The alkylating agents are active agents in a number of adult tumours and are used extensively in some of the haematological malignancies. Early studies with melphalan (M) and predisone (P) either with or without IFN (see chapter on myeloma) suggested that standard dose MP could be given together with IFN-alpha and that the response rates were increased from around 50% to 75%, indicating an at least additive antitumour effect. In one recent study [9] in small numbers of patients response rates of 68% and 95% for MP and MP plus IFN-alpha2a, respectively, were described with significant improvements in relapse-free and overall survivals. A possible explanation for this effect was sought by examining the pharmacokinetics of melphalan in combination with IFN [10]. Peak plasma levels and area under the time concentration curve (AUC) were lower when M was given 5 hours after IFN and the authors suggested that the improved antitumour effect of the combination was likely to be due to increased alkylating activity induced by the IFN.

A phase I study [11] recently determined that it was possible to administer cyclophosphamide at a dose of 150 mg/m^2/day for 5 days together with 3 mU/m^2 of IFN-alpha2b given subcutaneously (SC), initially daily for 5 days and then 3 times per week. Another study [12] has confirmed the feasibility of this approach in patients with favourable lymphoma and suggested that this might prove useful as induction therapy for these patients. As reviewed in another chapter of this monograph, similar studies have been carried out with chlorambucil plus IFN-alpha but it is as yet not clear whether the remission rates are improved. The results of a number of randomised clinical trials designed to determine if IFN has a role, in combination with chemotherapy, in the management of lymphoma patients, are eagerly awaited.

Anti-Metabolites

The anti-metabolites are chemotherapeutic agents which resemble important normal metabolites. They interfere at critical points in biochemical pathways by acting as false

Table 1. *In vitro* studies of the anti-metabolites plus the IFNs

Anti-metabolite	IFN subtype	Cell line	Effect	Reference
FUdR	β	Human colon cancer cells	synergism	Esgro et al. [14]
5FU	γ α/β	MCA 38 HL-60	synergism γ>>α/β no synergism for MCA 38 & IFN α/β	Elias and Crissman [15]
5FU	α	HL-60	synergism ⇑ FdUMP accumulation	Elias and Sandoval [16]
5FU & MTX	α/β/γ	Human gastric & pancreatic cells	β/γ most effective	Kimoto [17,18]
5FU & Ara C	γ	Human genito-urinary cancer cell lines	β/γ most effective	Yamamoto et al. [19]
5FU	γ	HT-29	synergism	Le et al. [20]
6 TG	α	HL-60 NK cells	synergism when pre-treated with 6 TG increase in NK cell mediated cytotoxicity	Tan et al. [21]
5FU	γ	KM 12c KM 12^r	additive no effect	Morikawa et al. [22-24]

5FU = 5 fluorouracil; MTX = methotrexate; Ara C = cytosine arabinoside; 6 TG = 6 thioguanine

substrates for or inhibiting the actions of enzymes essential for cellular proliferation. The enzymes most usually inhibited are those involved in RNA or DNA synthesis. Antimetabolites can, therefore, directly or indirectly cause nucleotide depletion and thus tend to be cell-cycle specific. It is this cell-cycle specificity which not only accounts for their cytotoxic effects against neoplastic cells but also their toxicity to normal tissues with a high proliferative capacity such as the bone marrow and gastrointestinal tract. Table 1 summarises the *in vitro* studies of the IFNs plus anti-metabolites. These data clearly demonstrate that in most experimental systems there is an additive or synergistic effect of combining these 2 classes of anticancer agents. One mechanism for the resistance of tumour cells to 5FU is an increase in the levels of the target enzyme thymidylate synthetase (TS). Chu et al. [13] were able to demonstrate that 5FU alone caused a 3-fold increase in TS levels, the combination of 5 FU and IFN-gamma suppressed this rise and prevented the development of resistance.

A perusal of the data presented in Table 1 demonstrates that IFN-gamma appears to give the best synergism with the antimetabolites, however, low concentrations (50-100 U/ml) of mixtures of IFN-gamma and IFN-alpha/beta were more effective than single IFN species [17]. This author also reported that anti-metabolites administered first, followed by IFN, was optimal but others have suggested that IFN pretreatment increased sensitivity to 5FU by enhancing the accumulation of FdUMP [16,25]. FdUMP is one of the active metabolites of 5FU which interferes with DNA

Table 2. Phase I/II clinical trials of 5FU plus IFN in colorectal carcinoma patients

5FU dose/schedule	IFN subtype	IFN dose	Toxicity	Results	Reference
750 mg/m^2/day x 5 continuous infusion	α2b	6,9,12,15,18 mU weekly SC	fatigue MTD 15-18 mU	56% OR	Wadler et al. [27]
750 mg/m^2/day x 5 continuous infusion 1 week rest & then 750 mg/m^2 weekly	α2a	9 mU x3/week SC	myelosuppression diarrhoea	76% OR	Wadler et al. [28]
500 mg/m^2/day x 5	γ	500 μg/day IM	malaise, fever, anorexia	2/29 PR	Ajani et al. [29]
250- 500 mg/m^2/day x 5 days continuous infusion	α2b	20 mU/m^2 IV or 5 mU/m^2 SC	unacceptable tolerable	no responses	Clark et al. [30]

MTD = maximum tolerable dose; OR = overall response rate; PR = partial response rate; SC = subcutaneous; IV = intravenous; IM = intramuscular

synthesis. This synergistic effect can be abrogated by thymidine and the synergy was greatest with FdUrd, which is preferentially metabolised to FdUMP.

It is unclear from these *in vitro* results which schedule is likely to be the most effective. Scheduling will probably be of critical importance *in vivo* where toxicity to normal cells must also be considered. IFN given after 5FU may also increase the antitumour effects of the combination by augmenting the immune response to the tumour [26]. Recently, a number of phase I/II studies have been reported which indicate that there may well be clinical synergy between 5FU and the IFNs with acceptable toxicity (Table 2). An alternative hypothesis, other than biochemical modulation, to explain the increased antitumour effects of these combinations has recently been put forward. Detailed pharmacokinetics of 5FU when given combined with IFN-alpha have shown that the AUC is substantially increased compared to that with 5FU alone (proceedings of the second European Interferon symposium, Hannover, Germany, February 1991). Phase III studies are currently in progress to confirm this in a randomised setting and to establish whether these combinations have a beneficial effect upon quality of life and duration of survival.

The Vinca Alkaloids

Vinblastine has been regarded as one of the only active chemotherapeutic agents in metastatic renal cell carcinoma. Response rates of between 10% and 15% have been reported in a large number of patients. Combinations of IFN and vinblastine (VBL) have been studied in phase I/II studies [31-35]. The MTDs for prolonged administration are 10 mU/m^2 x3/week and 0.1 mg/kg every 3 weeks for IFN and VBL, respectively. Thirty-one of the 114 patients (27%) treated in these studies responded. As reviewed in one of these papers [31], the response rate to IFN alone is 14% in 399 evaluable patients and 28% in 84 patients given the combination. Thus the combination of IFN and VBL may be more active than each agent used on its own, although a randomised trial would be necessary to confirm this. These data compare with the spontaneous regression rate of 7% seen when an initial surveillance policy is adopted [36].

Dacarbazine

A large number of phase II studies of single-agent dacarbazine in patients with metastatic melanoma have been conducted [37]. In over 300 patients the overall response rate is 11%. These data give the impression that the regimens which employ higher and more intensive treatment schedules may produce higher response rates. An overview of the published literature for dacarbazine [38] included some 1133 patients with metastatic melanoma of whom 239 (21%) responded. Only 1-2% of these patients have durable remissions and the median duration of all responses is only 5 to 6 months. McCleod and colleagues [39] administered IFN-alpha2a at a dose of 3 mU IM from days 1 to 3 and then 9 mU from days 4 to 70. This schedule was employed in order to induce tachyphylaxis with the lower dose with aim of improving tolerance for the higher dose of IFN. The dacarbazine was given in escalating doses of 200, 400 and 800 mg/m^2 IV every 3 weeks. Following this induction phase, the IFN was continued on a 3 times per week schedule. Of 43 patients entered, 6 (14%) achieved a complete and 7 (16%) a partial remission. At the time of reporting, 5 (12%) of the CR patients remained disease free at 9+ to 18+ months. Similar data have been reported by an American group [40] and the former group are now conducting a randomised trial comparing dacarbazine alone with the combination of dacarbazine with IFN-alpha2a.

Cisplatinum

The IFNs have no significant antitumour activity in non-small cell lung cancer [41,42]. Synergism between cisplatinum and IFN-alpha have, however, been demonstrated in 3 human non-small cell lung cancer xenografts [43]. These data led to the conduct of a phase II study of 3 or 5 mU of IFN-alpha2b x3/week starting 1 week before cisplatinum 100 mg/m^2 and then given every 4 weeks. Eighteen of 60 patients responded (30%, 95% confidence intervals 18-42%) with a median duration of 4.8 months (3-23+ months). Probability of response appeared to be dependent on histological subtype with 46%, 25% and 17% of squamous cell, adenocarcinoma and large cell responding respectively. Toxicity was not substantially increased with the possible exception of nausea and vomiting which was apparently worse than with single-agent cisplatinum. The authors concluded that this combination warranted further evaluation in a randomised trial of cisplatinum either with or without IFN, where quality of life and survival would be endpoints. These data suggest that combining cisplatinum with IFN may be a valid approach in tumour types which are responsive to cisplatinum. Perhaps combining IP cisplatinum and IFN would increase response rates in ovarian carcinoma where both agents have been shown to be active [44].

Miscellaneous Drugs

The alpha-IFNs have shown substantial effects in patients with myeloproliferative diseases. However, haematological control occurs relatively slowly and chronic toxicity often limits the dose and duration of therapy. Thus, the combination of IFN with a chemotherapeutic agent which is also active in these diseases is an attractive proposition. The combination has the potential of allowing lower and therefore less toxic doses of IFN to be used and of achieving a more rapid haematological remission. Anger and coworkers [45] induced remissions in 9 CML patients in a median time of 12 days to the normalisation of blood counts. Induction therapy consisted of 6 mU/day of IFN-alpha2b given for 1 week followed by a further week at 3 mU/day in combination with 40 mg/kg/day of hydroxyurea given orally. Maintenance was 3 mU IFN x3/week plus 0.5 to 1.0 gm/day of hydroxyurea. Toxicity was no worse than would have been expected from each agent individually and no patient stopped therapy for this reason. Another agent commonly used in CML is 6 thioguanine (6-TG). 6-TG has been shown to synergise with IFNalpha2b in *in vitro* studies [21] and combinations of 6-TG and IFN would be worth exploring in the clinic.

Groghan et al. [46] conducted a phase I study of the combination of IFN-alpha2b and alpha-difluoromethylornithine (DFMO), the latter agent being an irreversible inhibitor of ornithine decarboxylase. DFMO has been shown to have activity against B16 melanoma cells as well as *in vitro* and *in vivo* activity against human melanoma. Seventeen patients received 4 or 6 grams of oral DFMO daily for 11 days and the IFN was given IM on the first 11 days of each 14-day cycle. Dose-limiting toxicity occurred in 3/3 patients given 6 gm DFMO and 9 mU/m^2 IFN-alpha2a. Doses recommended for phase II testing are 4 gm DFMO and 6 mU/m^2 IFN. Further stimulus for these studies was given by the fact that 3 of the 17 patients entered responded (1 CR, liver and 2 PR, soft tissue, lung).

Monoclonal Antibodies and Other Antigen-Targeted Therapies

The modulation of class I and II major histocompatability complex (MHC) antigens on tumour cells may play an important role in the immune recognition of these cells by the host. A number of studies have investigated the role of the IFNs in inducing or increasing the expression of these important molecules both *in vitro* and *in vivo*. Results demonstrate that either class I or II molecules may indeed be induced or their expression increased in a variety of tumour cell types including breast cancer, melanoma, insulinoma, myeloid leukaemia and squamous carcinomas [47-54]. Two studies suggested that in melanoma changes in expression of these antigens occur during tumorigenesis and that various patterns may be important in determining the prognosis [55,56]. Changes in T-cell responses occurred parallel to these alterations in MHC expression and it seemed that IFN-gamma was important in modulating these effects. These data suggest that combinations of IFN and the adoptive transfer of appropriately sensitised T lymphocytes (tumour infiltrating or cytotoxic T lymphocytes) might be a fruitful area of future clinical research.

As well as being able to increase MHC expression, the IFNs are capable of modulating the expression of tumour-associated antigens (TAA). This subject has recently been reviewed by Borden [57]. He discussed the possible role of using IFN to increase TAA expression *in vivo*, thus allowing improved localisation of monoclonal antibodies to tumour sites. A further advantage of this combination would be the ability of the IFN to stimulate the effectors of antibody-dependent cellular cytotoxicity.

Two studies have demonstrated that improved monoclonal antibody localisation can be achieved *in vivo*. The first [58] employed IFN-alpha2a in nude mice bearing WiDr xenografts and the ^{125}I monoclonal antibody B6.2F(ab')$_2$. The localisation of antibody ranged from 2.16% to 4.61% in untreated animals and was between 3.47% and 12.89% after therapy with IFN. Rosenblum and colleagues [59] studied 5 melanoma patients with ^{111}In-labelled 96.5 monoclonal antibodies in whom IFN-alpha (non-recombinant) was administered simultaneously. They demonstrated a 3-fold increase in tumour to blood ratios compared to 5 patients matched for sites of metastatic disease but not treated with IFN. An increase in the proportion of antibody localising to the tumour, resulting from a pretreatment with IFN, would improve the clarity of diagnostic images and also the therapeutic index of radiation therapy targeted with monoclonal antibodies.

Hormone Therapy

Some breast cancers express receptors for oestrogen and progestrogen and these tumours have a high probability of responding to hormone manipulation. Indeed there is, in general, a positive correlation between the level of receptor expression and the probability of response. It can therefore be surmised that measures designed to increase the level of receptor expression within the tumour might lead to an enhancement of subsequent hormone therapy. The IFNs have been clearly demonstrated to have no single-agent antitumour activity in patients with metastatic breast cancer. Two papers have examined the interaction between IFNs and the antioestrogen tamoxifen. Van den Berg et al. [60] were able to demonstrate marked induction of oestrogen receptor expression in the human breast cancer cell line ZR-75-1. This increased receptor expression resulted in enhanced cytotoxicity of these cells to tamoxifen. Jacobelli and colleagues [61] showed not only a similar effect with tamoxifen in CG-5 human breast cancer cells but also noted that IFN alone inhibited the growth-promoting effect of oestrogen on these cells. This effect was mediated via an inhibition of the binding of oestrogen to its receptor. These data have profound clinical implications and deserve further investigation in clinical trials.

Radiation Therapy and Hyperthermia

A number of laboratory studies [62-66] have suggested that the IFNs may have radiosensitising properties. A phase I study of combined radiation therapy and IFN-alpha2b was reported in 1986 [67]. Sixteen patients, mostly with lung and oesophagus carcinomas, were treated with standard radiotherapy 5 days each week plus 1 of 2 schedules of IFN-a2b. The first schedule involved SC IFN on 5 days per week and the second on Mondays, Wednesdays and Fridays. In neither schedule could the dose be escalated above 5 mU/m^2 per injection. On the 5 times per week schedule only 22% tolerated the planned IFN doses and only 44% the planned radiation treatments. Equivalent figures for the 3 times per week scheme were 100% and 80%, respectively. The authors suggested that the latter protocol should be used for further phase II and III testing. No clinical data have been reported to support the hypothesis that IFN is a radiosensitiser.
Hyperthermia has been demonstrated to induce regression of tumours in both experimental animal systems and man. The results have, however, not been dramatic, and therefore combinations of systemic therapy plus hyperthermia are beginning to be explored. Human lymphoblastoid IFN-$_{N1}$ was given daily by IM or IP injection 60 minutes prior to the local application of hyperthermia in nude mice bearing renal cell carcinoma xenografts [68]. Five of 10 mice so treated demonstrated a complete disappearance of tumour and in the other animals survival was prolonged. In this model, recombinant human IFN-gamma was ineffective probably because it is heat labile. The same interferon was investigated in a phase I study in combination with whole body hyperthermia [69]. One, 3 and 10 mU/m^2 of IFN were investigated and the dose recommended for phase II studies was 3 mU/m^2 given daily for 6 days in conjunction with hyperthermia to 40.5°C for 75 minutes. The toxicities of the IFN and whole body hyperthermia combination did not seem increased above what has been observed with each individual component. Two responses were seen in patients with follicular lymphoma and melanoma lasting 7 and 5 months, respectively.

Combinations with Other Cytokines

Interleukin-2 (IL-2) has been shown to produce responses in 20-30% of patients with metastatic melanoma and renal cell carcinoma, with 8-10% achieving CR. The original protocol devised at the National Cancer Institute of the USA by Dr. Rosenberg [70] prescribed that the IL-2 should be given at its MTD. This decision was based on experiments in mice which demonstrated a clear dose-response effect. In an attempt to improve the results, Rosenberg's group have studied IFN-alpha2a plus IL-2 in a phase I study [71]. Both cytokines were given IV every 8 hours and the MTDs were 6 and 4.5 mU/m^2 per injection. There was a trend for the probability of response to be higher at increasing dosages and 11 of 27 (41%) at the highest dose level responded. These authors suggested that this is a higher response rate than is seen with either IFN or IL-2 alone. Of course randomised trials will be required to establish this as fact.
The above approach does produce considerable toxicity and requires intensive patient support during therapy. Another group [72] have taken a different approach based on a phase I/II study of IL-2 alone given by subcutaneous injection [73]. In the study reported by Atzpodien and colleagues [72] IL-2 was given for 2 days at a dose of 9 mIU/m^2 SC every 12 hours followed by 6 weeks of 1.8 mU/m^2 SC 12-hourly on days 1 to 5. The IFN-alpha2b was administered at a dose of 5 mU/m^2 SC on days 1, 3 and 5 concurrently with the IL-2. Five of 14 evaluable patients with renal cell carcinoma (35%) and 1 of 7 with melanoma responded. Toxicity was acceptable and the therapy could be administered as in an outpatient setting. WHO grade I/II fevers, chills and malaise were almost universal but hypotension was mild. Respiratory distress occurred in 20 of 52 cycles and was of WHO grade III severity in 2 of these cycles. Of some interest, 19 of 32 pa-

tients had thyroid dysfunction which "usually resolved within 4 weeks after completing therapy". Although the study by Atzpodien et al. [72] is of some considerable interest, it is unclear how they arrived at the doses of interferon and IL-2 used. No phase I study has been reported which has determined either MTD or the optimum immunomodulatory doses of the combination given by this schedule. The use of SC IL-2 was reported by the same authors [73] in what they called a phase II study. Unfortunately, the study design was such that we are still unaware of what the MTD, optimum immunomodulatory dose or probability of response of SC administered IL-2 is.

Based on the results of a phase I study [74] Krigel et al. [75] have conducted a phase II study of the combination of IL-2 and recombinant human IFN-beta in patients with renal cell carcinoma. Twenty-four patients were treated with bolus IV injections of the 2 cytokines 3 times per week at doses of 5 m Cetus U/m^2 of IL-2 and 6 mU/m^2 of IFN-beta. The major toxicities consisted of chronic fatigue, arthralgias, weight loss and depression. The haemodynamic toxicity and capillary leakage seen with high-dose IL-2 protocols were not common with this scheme. Six of 22 evaluable patients responded (27.2%; 95% confidence intervals 8.7% to 45.9%), with 5 of these responses occurring in the 10 patients who had undergone a prior nephrectomy. As has been observed with other IL-2 protocols, the responses can be of long duration with 3 of the 6 remissions continuing for longer than 18 months. Of interest was the fact that there was a positive correlation between the induction of NK and LAK activity and the probability of response in these patients.

In a phase I study Redman et al. [76] gave IL-2 as a continuous infusion daily for 5 days and simultaneously administered the IFN-gamma as 5 daily IM injections. The maximum tolerable doses were 1.0 m Cetus U/m^2/d for IL-2 and 0.5 mg/m^2/d of IFN-gamma. These doses were recommended for phase II studies despite the fact that the doses which optimally stimulated LAK cell generation were 1.0 mU/m^2/d and 0.25 mg/m^2/d of IL-2 and interferon gamma, respectively. Dose-limiting toxicity was pulmonary consisting of the development of rhales and dyspnoea. Although it has been suggested that interferon-gamma might protect endothelial cells from the damaging effects of LAK cells [77], the above combination did not allow higher doses of IL-2 to be administered. Another phase I study [78] using sequential IFN-gamma and IL-2 did appear to demonstrate that toxicity in the form of hypotension and capillary leakage was reduced by the prior administration of IFN-gamma.

The above data are the first from studies designed to examine combinations of cytokines. It is already clear that dosing, scheduling and routes of administration will be critical in determining the degree of toxicity induced and probably the potential of inducing anti-tumour effects.

Conclusions

The majority of clinical studies discussed above are of phase I or II design. They give a clear indication of the feasibility and potential of combining the IFNs with other modalities of cancer therapy. The coming years will hopefully begin to define the role that this approach will have in the overall management of patients with advanced cancer as the results of carefully designed phase III studies become available.

REFERENCES

1 Balkwill FR: Interferons. In: Cytokines in Cancer Therapy. Oxford University Press, Oxford 1989 pp 8
2 Balkwill FR: Interferons. Lancet 1989 (i):1060-1063
3 Yoneda K, Yamamoto T, Osaki T: Influence of interferon on adriamycin uptake of cultured tumour cells. Int J Cancer 1989 (44):483-488
4 Sarosy GA et al: Phase I study of α-2-interferon plus doxorubicin in patients with solid tumors. Cancer Res 1986 (46):5368-5371
5 Creagan ET et al: Phase I study of recombinant leukocyte A interferon (IFN-α2A, Roferon A) with doxorubicin in advanced malignant disease. Cancer 1989 (64):1034-1037
6 Green MD et al: Phase I trial of escalating doses of doxorubicin administered concurrently with α2-interferon. Cancer Res 1988 (48):2574-2578
7 Muss HB, Welander C, Caponera A et al: Interferon and doxorubicin in renal cell carcinoma. Cancer Treat Rep 1985 (60):721-722
8 Eksborg S, Mattson K: Pharmacokinetics of epirubicin in man. Non-influence of α-interferon. Med Oncol Tumor Pharmacother 1988 (5):131-133
9 Montuoro A, De Rosa L, De Blasio A, et al: Alpha-2a-interferon/melphalan/predisone versus melphalan/predisone in previously untreated patients with multiple myeloma. Br J Haematol 1991 (76):365-368
10 Ehrsson H, Eksborg S, Wallin I, et al: Oral melphalan pharmacokinetics: influence of interferon-induced fever. Clin Pharmacol Ther 1990 (47):86-90
11 Durie BGM, Clouse L, Braich T, et al: Interferon-α2b-cyclophosphamide combination studies: *in vitro* and phase I-II clinical results. Sem Oncol 1986 (13):84-88
12 Ozer H, Anderson JR, Peterson BA, et al: Combination trial of subcutaneous interferon-alpha-2b and oral cyclophosphamide in favourable histology non Hodgkin's lymphoma. Invest New Drugs 1987 (5 suppl):S27-33
13 Chu E, Zinn S, Allegra C: Mechanisms of interaction of gamma-interferon and 5-fluorouracil in a human colon cancer cell line (H630). Proc AACR 1990 (31): 420
14 Esgro JJ, Killion JJ, Fidler IJ: Modulation of the antiproliferative effect of floxuridine by interferon-beta against human colon carcinoma cells. Proc AACR 1990 (31): 425
15 Elias L, Crissman HA: Interferon effects upon adenocarcinoma 38 and HL-60 cell lines: antiproliferative responses and synergistic interactions with halogenated pyrimidine antimetabolites. Cancer Res 1988 (48):4868-4873
16 Elias L, Sandoval JM: Interferon effects upon fluorouracil metabolism by HL-60 cells. Biochem Biophys Res Comm 1989 (163):867-874
17 Kimoto Y: Combined effect of interferons alpha, beta and gamma on tumor growth in vitro. Gan to Kagaku Ryoho [6T8] 1986 (13):302-307
18 Kimoto Y: Antitumor effects of interferons with chemotherapeutic agents. Gan to Kagaku Ryoho [6T8] 1986 (13):293-301
19 Yamamoto Y, Tanaka H, Namba M: Potentiation of cytotoxic effects of anticancer drugs on human genitourinary neoplastic cells by recombinant gamma interferon. Gan to Kagaku Ryoho [6T8] 1987 (14):699-705
20 Le J, Yip Y, Vilcek J: Cytolytic activity of interferon gamma and its synergism with 5-fluorouracil. Int J Cancer 1984 (34):495-500
21 Tan YY, Epstein LB, Armstrong RD: In vitro evaluation of 6 TG and IFNα as a therapeutic combination in HL-60 and natural killer cells. Cancer Res 1989 (49):4431-4434
22 Morikawa K, Fidler IJ: Heterogenous response of human colon cancer cells to the cytostatic and cytotoxic effects of recombinant human cytokines. J Biol Resp Mod 1989 (8):206-218
23 Morikawa K, Fan D, Denkins YM et al: Mechanisms of combined effects of γ-interferon and 5-fluorouracil on human colon cancers implanted into nude mice. Cancer Res 1989 (49):799-805
24 Morikawa K, Morikawa R, Killion JJ, et al: Isolation of human carcinoma cells for resistance to a single interferon associated with a cross-resistance to multiple recombinant interferons: α, β and γ. JNCI 1990 (82): 517-522
25 Killion JJ, Fishback R, Littleton T, et al: The antiproliferative activity of fluorodeoxyuridine and interferon alpha against cultured human colon carcinoma cells depends upon the sequence of treatment. Proc AACR 1990 (31):425
26 D'Atri S, Fuggetta MP, Giganti G, et al: Comparative studies between in vitro and in vivo effects of human beta-interferon on natural killer activity and its relevance to immunochemotherapy. Cancer Immunol Immunother 1988 (27):163-170
27 Wadler S, Goldman M, Lyver A, et al: Phase I trial of 5-fluorouracil and recombinant α_{2a}-interferon in patients with advanced colorectal carcinoma. Cancer Res 1990 (50):2056-2059
28 Wadler S, Schwartz EL, Goldman M, et al: Fluorouracil and recombinant alfa-2a-interferon: an active regimen against advanced colorectal carcinoma. J Clin Oncol 1989 (7):1769-1775
29 Ajani JA, Rios AA, Ende K, et al: Phase I and II studies of the combination of recombinant human interferon-gamma and 5-fluorouracil in patients with advanced colorectal carcinoma. J Biol Response Mod 1989 (8):140-146
30 Clark PI, Slevin ML, Reznek RH et al: Two randomised phase II trials of intermittent intravenous versus subcutaneous alpha-2 interferon alone (trial 1) and in combination with 5-fluorouracil (trial 2) in advanced colorectal cancer. Int J Colon Dis 1987 (2):26-29
31 Rizzo M, Bartoletti R, Selli C, et al: Interferon alpha-2a and vinblastine in the treatment of metastatic renal carcinoma. Eur J Urol 1989 (16):271-277
32 Schornagel JH, Verweij J, ten Bokkel Huinink WW et al: Phase II study of recombinant interferon alpha-2a and vinblastine in advanced renal cell carcinoma. J Urol 1989 (142):253-256
33 Bergerat J-P, Herbrecht R, Dufour P, et al: Combination of recombinant interferon alpha-2a and

vinblastine in advanced renal cell cancer. Cancer 1988 (62):2320-2324
34 Trump DL, Ravdin PM, Borden EC, et al: Interferon-alpha-n1 and continuous infusion vinblastine for treatment of advanced renal cell carcinoma. J Biol Response Mod 1990 (9):108-111
35 Kellokumpu-Lehtinen P., Nordman E. (1990). Recombinant interferon-alpha 2a and vinblastine in advanced renal cell cancer: a clinical phase I-II study. J. Biol. Response Mod. 9:439-444
36 Oliver RTD, Nethersell ABW, Bottomley JM: Unexplained spontaneous regression and alpha-interferon as treatment for metastatic renal cell carcinoma. Br J Urol 1989 (63):128-131
37 Goldstein D, Laszlo J, Rudnick S: Interferon therapy in cancer. In: Oldham RK (ed) Principles of Cancer Biotherapy. Raven Press Ltd, New York, 1987 p 247
38 Comis RL: DTIC (NSC-45388) in malignant melanoma: a perspective. Cancer Treat Rep 1976 (60):165-176
39 McCleod GRC, Thomson DB, Hersey P: Recombinant interferon alfa-2a in advanced malignant melanoma: A phase I-II study in combination with DTIC. Int J Cancer 1987 (suppl 1):31-35
40 Kirkwood JM, Ernstoff MS, Giuliano A: Interferon alpha-2a and dacarbazine in melanoma. JNCI 1990 (82):1062-1068
41 Grunberg SM, Kempf RA, Itri LM et al: Phase II study of recombinant alpha interferon in the treatment of advanced non-small cell lung carcinoma. Cancer Treat Rep 1985 (69):1031-1032
42 Olesen BK, Ernst P, Nissen MH et al: Recombinant interferon A therapy of small cell and squamous cell carcinoma of the lung. A phase II study. Eur J Cancer Clin Oncol 1987 23:987-989
43 Carmichael J, Fergusson RJ, Wolf CR et al: Augmentation of cytotoxicity of chemotherapy by human alpha-interferon in human non-small cell lung cancer xenografts. Cancer Res 1986 (46):4916-4920
44 Berek J, Hacker N, Lichtenstein A et al: Intraperitoneal recombinant α-interferon for salvage immunotherapy in stage III epithelial ovarian cancer. Cancer Res 1985 (45):4447-4453
45 Anger B, Porzsolt F, Leichtle R, et al: A phase I/II study of recombinant interferon alpha 2a and hydroxyurea for chronic myeloid leukemia. Blut 1989 (58):275-278
46 Croghan MK, Booth A, Meyskens FL: A phase I trial of recombinant interferon-α and α-difluoromethylornithine in metastatic melanoma. J Biol Response Mod 1988 (7):409-415
47 Calvo F, Jabrane N, Faille A, et al: Quantitative modifications of major histocompatibility complex (MHC) antigens by recombinant gamma interferon in two human breast cancer cell lines. Int J Immunopharmacol 1987 (9):459-468
48 van Vliet E, Molenaar JL, Tuk CW et al: Recombinant gamma interferon induces class II major histocompatibility complex antigens on insulinoma cells. Tissue Antigens 1987 (29):195-200
49 Alonso MC, Navarrete C, Salana R et al: Modulation of the expression of HLA class II antigens by gamma interferon and phorbol ester TPA on myeloid leukaemia cells. J Immunogenet 1980 (13):255
50 Gross N, Beck D, Farre S, Carrel S: In vitro antigenic modulation of human neuroblastoma cells induced by IFN-G, retinoic acid and dibutyl cyclic AMP. Int J Cancer 1987 (39):521-529
52 Kameyama K, Tone T, Eto H et al: Recombinant gamma interferon induces HLA-DR expression on squamous cell carcinomas, trichilemmoma, adenocarcinoma cell lines and cultured human keratinocytes. Arch Dermatol Res 1987 (269):161-166
53 Balkwill FR, Stevens MH, Griffin DB et al: Interferon gamma regulates HLA-Dr expression on solid tumours *in vivo*. Eur J Cancer Clin Oncol 1987 (23):101-106
54 Carrington MN, Chedid M, Ting JP-Y, Ward FE: Differential expression of the HLA-DR genes in various melanoma cells treated with interferon gamma; methylation of the HLA-DR alpha gene in these cell lines is not correlated with expression. Hum Immunol 1987 (18):151-161
55 Guerry D, Alexander MA, Elder DE, Herlyn MF: Interferon-gamma regulates the T cell response to precursor nevi and biologically early melanoma. J Immunol 1987 (139):305-312
56 Ruiter DJ, Brocker E-B, Ferrone S: Expression and susceptibility to modulation by interferons of HLA class I and II antigens on melanoma cells. Immunohistochemical analysis and clinical relevance. J Immunogenet 1986 (13):229-234
57 Borden EC: Augmented tumor-associated antigen expression by interferons. JNCI 1988 (80):148-149
58 Greiner JW, Guadagni F, Noguchi P et al: Recombinant interferon enhances monoclonal antibody targeting to carcinoma lesions in vivo. Science 1987 (235):895-898
59 Rosenblum MG, Lamki LM, Murray JL et al: Interferon induced changes in pharmacokinetics and tumor uptake of ^{111}In-labelled antimelanoma antibody 96.5 in melanoma patients. JNCI 1988 (80):160-165
60 Van den Berg HW, Leahey WJ, Lynch M et al: Recombinant human interferon alpha increases oestrogen receptor expression in human breast cancer cells (ZR-75-1) and sensitivities to the anti-proliferative effects of tamoxifen. Br J Cancer 1987 (55):255-257
61 Iacobelli S, Natoli C, Arno E et al: An antiestrogenic action of interferons in human breast cancer cells. Anticancer Res 1986 (6):1391-1394
62 Dritschilo A, Mossman K, Gray M, Sreeralsan T: Potentiation of radiation injury by interferon. Am J Clin Oncol 1982 (5):79-82
63 Nederman T, Benedlktsson G: Effects of interferon on growth rate and radiation sensitivity of cultured human glioma cells. Acta Radiol Oncol 1982 (21):231-234
64 Gould MN, Kakria R, Olson S, Borden E: Radiosensitisation of human bronchogenic carcinoma cells by interferon beta. J Interferon Res 1984 (4):123-128

65 Namba M, Yamamoto S, Tanaka H et al: Potentiation of cytotoxic effects of anticancer drugs or cobalt-60 gamma rays by interferon on neoplastic cells. Cancer 1984 (54):2262-2267

66 Lvovsky E, Mossman K, Levy H, Dritschilo A: Response of mouse tumor to interferon inducer and radiation. Int J Radiat Oncol Biol Phys 1985 (11):1721-1725

67 Torrisi J, Berg C, Harler K et al: Phase I combined modality clinical trial of alpha-2-interferon and radiotherapy. Int J Radiat Oncol Biol Phys 1986 (12):1453-1456

68 Onishi T, Machida T, Mori Y et al: Hyperthermia with simultaneous administration of interferon using established human renal cell carcinoma heterotransplanted nude mice. Br J Urol 1989 (63):227-232

69 Robins HI, Sielaff KM, Storer B et al: Phase I trial of human lymphoblastoid interferon with whole body hyperthermia in advanced cancer. Cancer Res 1989 (49):160901615

70 Rosenberg SA, Lotze MT, Yang JC et al: Experience with the use of high-dose interleukin-2 in the treatment of 652 cancer patients. Ann Surg 1989 (210):474-484

71 Rosenberg SA, Lotze MT, Yang JC et al: Combination therapy with interleukin-2 and alpha interferon for the treatment of patients with advanced cancer. J Clin Oncol 1989 (7):1863-1874

72 Atzpodien J, Körfer A, Franks CR et al: Home therapy with recombinant human interleukin-2 and interferon-α2b in advanced human malignancies. Lancet 1990 (335):1509-1512

73 Atzpodien J, Körfer A, Evers P et al: Low-dose subcutaneous interleukin-2 in advanced human malignancy: a phase II outpatient study. Mol Biother 1990 (2):18-26

74 Krigel RL, Padaric-Shaller KA, Rudolph AR et al: A phase I study of recombinant interleukin-2 plus recombinant β interferon. Cancer Res 1988 (48):3875-3881

75 Krigel RL, Padaric-Shaller KA, Rudolph AR et al: Renal cell carcinoma: treatment with recombinant interleukin-2 plus beta interferon. J Clin Oncol 1990 (8):460-467

76 Redman BG, Flaherty L, Chou T-H et al: A phase I trial of recombinant interleukin-2 combined with recombinant interferon-gamma in patients with cancer. J Clin Oncol 1990 (8):1269-1276

77 Renkonen R, Ristimäki A, Häyry P: Interferon-gamma protects human endothelial cells from lymphokine activated killer cell mediated lysis. Eur J Immunol 1988 (18):1839-1842

78 Wagstaff J, Vermorken JB, Schwartzmann G: A progress report of a phase I study of interferon gamma and interleukin-2 and some comments on the mechanism of the toxicity due to interleukin-2. Cancer Treat Rev 1989 (16 suppl A):105-109

ESO Monographs

Series Editor: U. Veronesi

L. Denis, Antwerp (Ed.)

The Medical Management of Prostate Cancer II

1991. VII, 100 pp. 16 figs. 23 tabs. Hardcover ISBN 3-540-53443-1

J. Hildebrand, Free University of Brussels (Ed.)

Neurological Adverse Reactions to Anticancer Drugs

1990. VII, 99 pp. 8 figs. 15 tabs. Hardcover ISBN 3-540-53263-3

L. Domellöf, Örebro (Ed.)

Drug Delivery in Cancer Treatment III

Home Care – Symptom Control, Economy, Brain Tumours

1990. VIII, 125 pp. 34 figs. 38 tabs. Hardcover ISBN 3-540-52951-9

A. Goldhirsch, Lugano (Ed.)

Endocrine Therapy of Breast Cancer IV

1990. VIII, 97 pp. 19 figs. 40 tabs. Hardcover ISBN 3-540-52961-6

L. Tomatis, Lyon (Ed.)

Air Pollution and Human Cancer

1990. VII, 86 pp. 7 figs. 10 tabs. Hardcover ISBN 3-540-52901-2

E. J. Freireich, University of Texas, Houston, TX (Ed.)

New Approaches to the Treatment of Leukemia

1990. VII, 193 pp. 37 figs. 36 tabs. Hardcover ISBN 3-540-52261-1

R. Mertelsmann, Freiburg (Ed.)

Lymphohaematopoietic Growth Factors in Cancer Therapy

1990. VII, 90 pp. 8 figs. 14 tabs. Hardcover ISBN 3-540-53086-X

S. Monfardini, Aviano (Ed.)

The Management of Non-Hodgkin's Lymphomas in Europe

1990. VIII, 92 pp. 13 figs. 12 tabs. Softcover ISBN 3-540-52297-2

J. C. Holland, New York; **R. Zittoun**, Paris (Eds.)

Psychosocial Aspects of Oncology

1990. VIII, 142 pp. 3 figs. Hardcover ISBN 3-540-51947-5

A. Breit, Technical University of Munich (Ed.-in-Chief)

Magnetic Resonance in Oncology

A. L. Baert, R. Felix, R. Musumeci, W. Semmler and G. Sze (Co-Eds.)

1990. XIII, 173 pp. 147 figs. 7 tabs. Hardcover ISBN 3-540-51054-0

A. B. Miller, University of Toronto, Ont. (Ed.)

Diet and the Aetiology of Cancer

1989. VII, 73 pp. 2 figs. Hardcover ISBN 3-540-50681-0

F. Cavalli, Bellinzona (Ed.)

Endocrine Therapy of Breast Cancer III

1989. VII, 65 pp. 26 figs. 7 tabs. Hardcover ISBN 3-540-50819-8

L. Domellöf, Örebro (Ed.)

Drug Delivery in Cancer Treatment II

Symptom Control, Cytokines, Chemotherapy

1989. VII, 107 pp. 31 figs. Hardcover ISBN 3-540-51055-9

L. Denis, Antwerp (Ed.)

The Medical Management of Prostate Cancer

1988. IX, 98 pp. 8 figs. Hardcover ISBN 3-540-18627-1

B. Winograd, Amsterdam; **M. Peckham**, London; **H. M. Pinedo**, Amsterdam (Eds.)

Human Tumour Xenografts in Anticancer Drug Development

1988. XV, 143 pp. 37 figs. Hardcover ISBN 3-540-18638-7

L. Domellöf, Örebro (Ed.)

Drug Delivery in Cancer Treatment

1987. VII, 99 pp. Hardcover ISBN 3-540-18459-7

J. F. Smyth, Edinburgh (Ed.)

Interferons in Oncology

Current Status and Future Directions

1987. VII, 70 pp. Hardcover ISBN 3-540-18019-2

F. Cavalli, Bellinzona (Ed.)

Endocrine Therapy of Breast Cancer

Concepts and Strategies

1986. VII, 120 pp. Hardcover ISBN 3-540-16959-8

In preparation:

P. A. Jr. Bunn, University of Colorado, Denver, CO (Ed.)

Current Topics in Lung Cancer

1991. Approx. 82 pp. 1 fig. 24 tabs. Hardcover ISBN 3-540-54301-5

Springer-Verlag
Berlin Heidelberg New York London Paris Tokyo Hong Kong Barcelona

www.ingramcontent.com/pod-product-compliance
Lightning Source LLC
Chambersburg PA
CBHW061224240926
51846CB00006B/1347